MALARIA CONTROL DURING MASS POPULATION MOVEMENTS AND NATURAL DISASTERS

Peter B. Bloland and Holly A. Williams

Roundtable on the Demography of Forced Migration
Committee on Population

NATIONAL RESEARCH COUNCIL
OF THE NATIONAL ACADEMIES

and
Program on Forced Migration and Health at the
Mailman School of Public Health of
Columbia University

THE NATIONAL ACADEMIES PRESS
Washington, DC
www.nap.edu

THE NATIONAL ACADEMIES PRESS   500 Fifth Street, N.W.   Washington, DC 20001

NOTICE: The project that is the subject of this report was approved by the Governing Board of the National Research Council, whose members are drawn from the councils of the National Academy of Sciences, the National Academy of Engineering, and the Institute of Medicine. The members of the committee responsible for the report were chosen for their special competences and with regard for appropriate balance.

This study was supported by a grant to the National Academy of Sciences and the Mailman School of Public Health of Columbia University by the Andrew W. Mellon Foundation. Any opinions, findings, conclusions, or recommendations expressed in this publication are those of the authors and do not necessarily reflect the view of the organizations or agencies that provided support for this project.

Library of Congress Cataloging-in-Publication Data

Bloland, Peter B.
  Malaria control during mass population movements and natural disasters
/ Peter B. Bloland and Holly A. Williams ; [presented to] Roundtable on
the Demography of Forced Migration, Committee on Population and Program
on Forced Migration and Health, Mailman School of Public Health,
Columbia University.
     p. ; cm.
Includes bibliographical references.
  ISBN 0-309-08615-9 (pbk.)
  1. Malaria—Epidemiology. 2. Disaster medicine. 3. Emigration and
immigration—Health aspects.
  [DNLM: 1. Malaria—prevention & control. 2. Emigration and
Immigration. 3. Natural Disasters. 4. Relief Work. WC 765 B652m
2003] I. Williams, Holly A. II. Roundtable on the Demography of Forced
Migration. III. Joseph L. Mailman School of Public Health. Program on
Forced Migration and Health. IV. Title.
  RA644.M2 B566 2003
  614.5'32—dc21
                         2002151428

Suggested citation: National Research Council. (2003). *Malaria Control During Mass Population Movements and Natural Disasters.* Peter B. Bloland and Holly A. Williams. Roundtable on the Demography of Forced Migration. Committee on Population, Division of Behavioral and Social Sciences and Education and Program on Forced Migration and Health at the Mailman School of Public Health of Columbia University, Washington, DC: The National Academies Press.

Additional copies of this report are available from the National Academies Press, 500 Fifth Street, N.W., Lockbox 285, Washington, DC 20055; (800) 624-6242 or (202) 334-3313 (in the Washington metropolitan area); Internet, http://www.nap.edu

THE NATIONAL ACADEMIES
Advisers to the Nation on Science, Engineering, and Medicine

The **National Academy of Sciences** is a private, nonprofit, self-perpetuating society of distinguished scholars engaged in scientific and engineering research, dedicated to the furtherance of science and technology and to their use for the general welfare. Upon the authority of the charter granted to it by the Congress in 1863, the Academy has a mandate that requires it to advise the federal government on scientific and technical matters. Dr. Bruce M. Alberts is president of the National Academy of Sciences.

The **National Academy of Engineering** was established in 1964, under the charter of the National Academy of Sciences, as a parallel organization of outstanding engineers. It is autonomous in its administration and in the selection of its members, sharing with the National Academy of Sciences the responsibility for advising the federal government. The National Academy of Engineering also sponsors engineering programs aimed at meeting national needs, encourages education and research, and recognizes the superior achievements of engineers. Dr. Wm. A. Wulf is president of the National Academy of Engineering.

The **Institute of Medicine** was established in 1970 by the National Academy of Sciences to secure the services of eminent members of appropriate professions in the examination of policy matters pertaining to the health of the public. The Institute acts under the responsibility given to the National Academy of Sciences by its congressional charter to be an adviser to the federal government and, upon its own initiative, to identify issues of medical care, research, and education. Dr. Harvey V. Fineberg is president of the Institute of Medicine.

The **National Research Council** was organized by the National Academy of Sciences in 1916 to associate the broad community of science and technology with the Academy's purposes of furthering knowledge and advising the federal government. Functioning in accordance with general policies determined by the Academy, the Council has become the principal operating agency of both the National Academy of Sciences and the National Academy of Engineering in providing services to the government, the public, and the scientific and engineering communities. The Council is administered jointly by both Academies and the Institute of Medicine. Dr. Bruce M. Alberts and Dr. Wm. A. Wulf are chair and vice chair, respectively, of the National Research Council.

www.national-academies.org

v

Preface

In response to the need for more research on displaced persons, the Committee on Population developed the Roundtable on the Demography of Forced Migration in 1999. This activity, which is supported by the Andrew W. Mellon Foundation, provides a forum in which a diverse group of experts can discuss the state of knowledge about demographic structures and processes among people who are displaced by war and political violence, famine, natural disasters, or government projects or programs that destroy their homes and communities. The roundtable includes representatives from operational agencies, with long-standing field and administrative experience. It includes researchers and scientists with both applied and scholarly expertise in medicine, demography, and epidemiology. The group also includes representatives from government, international organizations, donors, universities, and nongovernmental organizations.

The roundtable is organized to be as inclusive as possible of relevant expertise and to provide occasions for substantive sharing to increase knowledge for all participants with a view toward developing cumulative facts to inform policy and programs in complex humanitarian emergencies. To this aim, the roundtable has held annual workshops on a variety of topics, including mortality patterns in complex emergencies, demographic assessment techniques in emergency settings, and research ethics among conflict-affected and displaced populations.

Another role for the roundtable is to serve as a promoter of the best research in the field. The field is rich in practitioners but is lacking a coherent body of research. In recent years a number of attempts to codify health policies and practices for the benefit of the humanitarian assistance community have been launched. The SPHERE Project—a collaboration of a large group of nongovernmental organizations—has produced a set of guidelines for public health interventions in emergency settings. The nongovernmental organization Médecins Sans Frontières has published a book entitled *Refugee Health: An Approach to Emergency Situations* (1997). In addition, a number of short-term training courses have been developed, including the Health Emergencies in Large Populations (HELP) course sanctioned by the International Committee of the Red Cross and the Public Health in Complex Emergencies course, which is partially funded by the U.S. Agency for International Development. All of these are intended to convey the "state of the art" to health care practitioners who serve refugees.

Yet the scientific basis for these currently recommended "best practices" is rarely presented along with the guidelines. And many of the current recommendations are based on older, perhaps even outdated, analyses and summaries of the literature. Furthermore, even when data are available, they are frequently inconsistent, unreliable, and spotty. Few of the currently recommended practices are based on scientifically valid epidemiological or clinical studies conducted among the refugee populations they are intended to benefit. Recognition of the need for a more evidence-based body of knowledge to guide the public health work practiced by the relief community has led to a widespread call for more epidemiological research. This was acted on by the World Health Organization, which formed an Advisory Group for Research in Emergency Settings.

In some sense the current wave of recommendations represents the end of a cycle of learning that began with the publication of a series of papers in the medical literature in the late 1980s. The data contained in those papers were originally generated during the period 1978-1986. But the world and the nature of forced migration have changed a great deal since then, and the relevance of those data can now be called into question. Therefore, the roundtable and the Program on Forced Migration and Health at the Mailman School of Public Health of Columbia University have commissioned a series of epidemiological reviews on priority public health problems for forced migrants that will update the state of knowledge. These occasional monographs will be individually authored documents presented to the roundtable and any recommendations or conclusions will be solely attributable to the authors. It is hoped these reviews will result in the formulation of newer and more scientifically sound public health practices and policies and will identify areas where new research is needed to guide the development of health care policy. Many of the monographs may represent newer areas of concern for which no summary information is available in the published literature.

The present monograph—on malaria control—is the first in this series. It provides a basic overview of the state of knowledge about the epidemiology of malaria and public health interventions and practices for controlling the disease in situations involving forced displacement and conflict. Other topics under consideration include reviews of current knowledge on diarrheal diseases, malnutrition (particularly micronutrient disorders), psychosocial issues, and reproductive health.

This report has been reviewed by individuals chosen for their diverse perspectives and technical expertise in accordance with procedures approved by the National Research Council's Report Review Committee. The purpose of this independent review was to provide candid and critical comments that would assist the institution in making the published monograph as accurate and as sound as possible. The review comments and draft manuscript remain confidential.

Ronald J. Waldman of Columbia University served as review coordinator for this report. We wish to thank the following individuals for their participation in the review of this report: Mary Ettling of the Office of Sustainable Development, Bureau for Africa, United States Agency for International Development, and Dominique Legros of Epi Centre, Médecins Sans Frontières, Paris.

Although the individuals listed above provided constructive comments and suggestions, it must be emphasized that responsibility for this monograph rests entirely with the authors.

We are also grateful to the staff and associates of the National Research Council. Ana-Maria Ignat assisted with the proofreading and formatting of the manuscript. Barbara Bodling O'Hare edited the volume. Christine McShane skillfully assisted with the editing and Yvonne Wise guided the manuscript through the publication process. Development and execution of this project occurred under the general guidance of Barney Cohen, director of the Committee on Population.

The authors, Peter B. Bloland and Holly A. Williams, work with the Malaria Epidemiology Branch in the Division of Parasitic Diseases, National Center for Infectious Diseases, Centers for Disease Control and Prevention in Atlanta, Georgia.

The authors also thank John Sexton, Ray Beach, Eric Noji, Brent Burkholder, Gail Stennies, and Paul Spiegel for their comments on a draft version of this report.

This series of monographs is being made possible by a special collaboration between the Roundtable on the Demography of Forced Migration of the National Academy of Sciences and the Program on Forced Migration and Health at the Mailman School of Public Health of Columbia University. We thank the Andrew W. Mellon Foundation for its continued support of the work of the roundtable and the program at Columbia. A special thanks is due Carolyn Makinson of the Mellon Foundation for her enthusiasm and significant expertise in the field of forced migration, which she has shared with the roundtable, and for her help in facilitating partnerships such as this.

Most of all, we are grateful to the authors of this report. We hope that this publication contributes to both better policy and better practice in the field.

Charles B. Keely
Chair, Roundtable on the Demography of Forced Migration

Ronald J. Waldman
Member, Roundtable on the Demography of Forced Migration

Holly E. Reed
Program Officer, Roundtable on the Demography of Forced Migration

Contents

MALARIA CONTROL DURING MASS POPULATION MOVEMENTS AND NATURAL DISASTERS

1

Introduction

In recent years, large-scale population movements in troubled areas of the world and the suffering associated with these displacements have caught the attention of the media. Often, the media's attention focuses on the political vulnerabilities of the uprooted populations, the turmoil that caused the displacement, the malnourished state of the displaced, and occasionally, communicable disease epidemics, such as cholera, that occur in such settings. Rarely is it noted, however, that such displacement often occurs in malarious areas and that malaria is frequently a primary cause of death in the displaced population. Nonetheless, humanitarian responses to these situations have rarely given malaria control activities the degree of emphasis and the level of resources that the burden of disease and death due to the disease would seem to demand. In the past, malaria control in complex emergencies was a relatively low-priority activity that was often disorganized, poorly conceived, and, ultimately, inadequate. The field-based practice of malaria control in complex emergencies typically did not reflect a thorough and current understanding of the disease and its contributing factors and failed to adequately capitalize on lessons learned from stable situations. More recently, with the attention given to malaria by global initiatives such as Roll Back Malaria (<*http://www.who.int/inf-fs/en/ InformationSheet02.pdf*>), there has been a noticeable increase in concern about the impact of malaria in complex emergencies and a desire to improve malaria control activities during mass population movements (Rowland and Nosten, 2001; <*http://www.who.int/inf-fs/en/InformationSheet07.pdf*>).

This is not to say that achieving effective malaria control is easy. Even among stable communities, the level of commitment and resources needed is substantial. As there is no simple "one size fits all" approach to malaria control, and in recognition of the multitude of factors influencing the potential success of any malaria control program, it becomes incumbent on those providing the services to base their decisions on the best practices available for the given situation. This, in turn, requires a familiarity with the technical aspects of malaria, an ability to obtain the information needed to make informed decisions, and a flexibility to match or adapt interventions to the local situation. An ability to facilitate effective communication and coordination among those involved (not just the relief community but the displaced and host communities as well) in order to develop an integrated plan of action is essential. Finally, adherence to best practices requires a commitment to address malaria with as much serious planning and forethought as are applied to the provision of water, sanitation, food, and shelter. In many situations the burden of disease and death attributable to malaria easily justifies this commitment.

This monograph is intended to provide humanitarian workers with a comprehensive review of those aspects of malaria control that are most relevant to designing and implementing a program in response to mass population movements. Where possible, field-based examples from complex emergencies have been used to illustrate different approaches, some successful and others not. The intent is not to present a "cookbook" for malaria control but rather to provide the relief generalist with an overview of proven or promising malaria control interventions and enough background information to make informed decisions or to facilitate the recognition of when outside expertise and advice are required. Effective malaria control during mass population movements is more likely to be achievable given a willingness to become informed and prepared beforehand; it is hoped that this report will assist relief organizations to become better prepared to deal with this potentially devastating disease.[1]

---

[1]Use of trade names throughout this monograph is for identification only and does not imply endorsement by the U.S. Public Health Service or the U.S. Department of Health and Human Services.

WHY MALARIA CONTROL IN EMERGENCY SITUATIONS?

Mass population movements are not a new phenomenon; they have resulted from wars and natural disasters since antiquity. During the past several years a large number of conflicts in diverse regions of the world have forced millions of civilians to flee their homes and seek refuge in other areas of their country or in neighboring countries. People have also been forced to leave their homes because of natural disasters such as floods or droughts leading to severe food shortages. Periods of major social or environmental change often cause a secondary migration in which people move to seek better economic opportunities.

In recent years many forced population movements have occurred in areas where malaria constitutes a substantial public health threat. The World Health Organization lists environmental disruption for agricultural or economic reasons, sociopolitical unrest, and migration as probable precipitating causes of the most serious malaria problems (World Health Organization, 1996a). Additionally, it has estimated that as many as one-third of malaria deaths in Africa occur in countries that have been affected by complex emergencies (Whyte, 2000).

Malaria occurs in over 90 countries worldwide, and 36 percent of the world's population lives in areas where there is risk of malaria transmission; 29 percent of the world's population lives in areas where malaria was once transmitted at low levels or not at all but where significant transmission has been reestablished. An additional 7 percent lives in areas where malaria has never been under meaningful control (World Health Organization, 1996a). Each year there are an estimated 200 million to 500 million clinical cases of malaria and 990,000 to 2 million deaths, the majority of the deaths occurring in sub-Saharan Africa. The magnitude of this burden of illness makes malaria one of the world's most important infectious diseases (World Health Organization, 1996a; Snow et al., 1999; Greenwood and Mutabingwa, 2002).

In certain epidemiological circumstances, malaria can be a devastating disease with high morbidity and mortality that deserves rapid and comprehensive response. In other settings, while malaria may not be an important cause of severe illness and death, it may have a more subtle public health impact through increased morbidity, loss of productivity, and exacerbation of other problems, such as anemia and malnutrition. In many malarious areas of the world, especially sub-Saharan Africa, the disease is ranked among the most frequent causes of morbidity and mortality among children and is often the leading cause of each. If this is the case for the stable host community, it is reasonable to expect that it will also be the case for a displaced population that finds itself in the midst of that host community. For a variety of reasons, malaria may actually be a far worse problem in the displaced population than it is in the surrounding community (Suleman, 1988).

Public health responses to mass population movements due to a complex emergency[2] or natural disaster typically represent a compromise between competing priorities and finite resources. Informed decisions, at times difficult ones, must be made as early as possible to define which components are most urgently needed and which should receive financial and logistical support. This is especially true during the initial emergency phase of a sudden or unexpected mass population movement. Adequate food, shelter, clean water, and sanitation are clear priorities (Toole and Waldman, 1990; Sphere Project, 2000). Responding to epidemics or the threat of epidemics due to diseases with high attack rates or high mortality (including malaria) is also a clear priority, especially in the case of diseases with an easily defined and practical intervention such as immunization. Defining the appropriate response for endemic diseases without a simple intervention, however, is far more difficult and may come down to a decision favoring what is operationally realistic over what is technologically possible.

Such is the case with designing an appropriate ongoing malaria control program. Factors such as the intensity of malaria transmission, the level of immunity in the population, the biology of the locally prevalent parasite and vector, and the ecology of the location can all influence the design of an integrated malaria control effort. While there are technological solutions to most of the uncertainties presented by these variables, many are expensive, complex, or unsustainable. Because of the potential for malaria to be a major cause of illness and death among displaced populations, decisions about what approaches to support and implement need to be made on the basis of a solid understanding of the disease, the local malaria situation, the political/economic context in which relief operations occur, and a familiarity with control options.

---

[2]Complex emergencies are generally defined as situations in which large civilian populations are exposed to war or civil strife, food shortages, and population displacement resulting in excess morbidity and mortality (Duffield, 1994; Palmer and Zwi, 1998; Goodhand and Hulme, 1999).

Provision of easily accessible and effective malaria therapy is an essential component of health care in areas where malaria transmission occurs, as well as in epidemic-prone areas and situations where populations are arriving from malaria-endemic areas. However, many agencies fail to make an effective transition from the initial stages in a complex emergency where the focus is on malaria case management, to the later stages where control activities should broaden to include both curative and preventive services. While malaria can certainly be an epidemic disease, with high attack rates and high mortality rates, its potential impact in nonepidemic settings should not be ignored.

Objectives of This Report

Any agency accepting responsibility for providing medical or public health services to a displaced population in or from an area where malaria transmission occurs will need to be prepared to deal effectively with malaria control. Similarly, organizations responding to public health needs following natural disasters or governments anticipating environmental disruption due to development projects must consider the possibility of increases in malaria transmission and the need for enhanced malaria control efforts on a temporary or permanent basis. Our objectives in this report are to describe in detail aspects that are most relevant to designing a malaria control program in response to a mass movement of people. The focus is primarily on situations of displacement, such as can occur with complex emergencies, natural disasters, or some development projects. The principles discussed here can also be applied to more stable nonemergency situations.

There is a growing body of evidence and literature that address malaria control in situations of mass population movement; however, much still needs to be better understood. Wherever possible, examples and experiences from displacement situations are given here. However, many interventions and programs that have been successfully evaluated in stable communities have not been satisfactorily evaluated among displaced populations. Nonetheless, these experiences may offer insights and lessons into approaches that could be modified to address the needs of displaced populations.

Making sound decisions regarding malaria control in any situation requires a familiarity with malaria itself, including the epidemiology of the disease; the life cycle of the parasite; and the interaction between parasite, human host, environment, and mosquito vector. On the other hand, the realities of addressing an evolving complex emergency argue strongly in favor of providing straightforward and practical advice. Further complicating the situation, any mass movement of people will also have implications for the host population. A basic tenet of humanitarian relief is that assistance should be offered to those in need in a refugee- or displacement-affected area, but this tenet is often forgotten or ignored due to constraints associated with lack of funding, poor access and utilization, and political sensitivities (Wilson, 1992). Health care and other essential services should be integrated, whenever possible, into the existing services and policies of the host population (Cromwell, 1988; Van Damme et al., 1998).

The intended audience for this monograph is primarily generalist relief workers who are in the position to develop, implement, and support disease control programs at the field, country, or home office level. While recommendations are provided that would be of use to clinical staff regarding the management of malaria, this paper is not intended as a handbook for action without first understanding the context of a situation. Approaches that may work in one setting may fail in another; decisions about which approaches are practical, logistically feasible, or economically justifiable in any given situation can only be made on a case-by-case basis. The intent is to (1) provide a basic technical background on malaria; (2) offer practical advice based on available evidence; and (3) where possible, provide field-based examples. Together, this information should help those involved in humanitarian relief efforts make reasonable policy and programmatic decisions that address the local malaria situation and the political realities in the field. Nonetheless, no written review can offer the quality of information provided by a consulting expert. To help the reader obtain qualified assistance, potential sources of technical assistance are also provided (see Appendix D). Addressing malaria in complex emergencies requires proper preparation and planning as well as adequate training for field personnel.

RECOMMENDATIONS

• Require training in the fundamentals of malaria control, including the basics of epidemiology, entomology, clinical and behavioral considerations, and political factors that affect the provision and receipt of malaria services.

• Develop generalized contingency plans to address malaria control pro-actively. Initially, these plans could be devised using existing information to reflect the malaria situation regionally (such as for Tropical sub-Saharan Africa, Southeast Asia, or Central Asia) and then modified as needed for specific local conditions (see Appendix D for information resources). These contingency plans should form the framework for developing a comprehensive and locally appropriate malaria control program.

• Be prepared to conduct a rapid initial assessment of the local malaria situation in order to be able to modify contingency plans as well as properly prioritize malaria control in relation to other locally relevant health needs.

• Provide or generate adequate financial resources for implementation of malaria control activities.

• Produce and implement a plan for monitoring and evaluating the effectiveness of the control program.

Why Malaria Control in Emergency Situations?
Key Points

• Mass population movements often occur in areas where malaria is transmitted.

• Given certain epidemiological conditions, malaria can be responsible for substantial levels of morbidity and mortality, especially in displaced populations.

• Effective malaria control, which is challenging in stable situations, becomes even more difficult in situations of displacement.

• Decisions about the most appropriate malaria control strategies to employ during a complex emergency are best made with an understanding of all the factors involved (epidemiological, entomological, clinical, behavioral, and political).

2

Malaria and Mobility—
A Brief History and Overview

Human mobility has had a tremendous effect on the global malaria situation. Among 20 countries with high risk of malaria transmission in the Americas, 16 have identified human mobility as a major cause of persistence of transmission (Pan American Health Organization, 1995). Migration has been associated with the spread of drug-resistant malaria in Africa and Southeast Asia and with dramatic change in the local epidemiology of malaria in Pakistan (Verdrager, 1986; Thimisarn et al., 1995; Kazmi and Pandit, 2001). In Kenya, seasonal movement of large numbers of workers from lowland areas to highland tea plantations has been associated with yearly epidemics (Malakooti et al., 1998; Shanks et al., 2000). Seasonal movement of migrant farm workers from Central and South America has been associated with outbreaks of local transmission of malaria in the United States (Zucker, 1996), raising concerns about the possibility of reestablishment of local transmission (Olliaro et al., 1996).

Even movements of individuals or small numbers of people can have an effect on the malaria situation in a given area, as evidenced by the outbreaks of local transmission in the United States (Zucker, 1996). Movements of large populations either into or out of malaria-endemic areas, however, have a much greater likelihood of disastrous consequences.

SPEED, DURATION, AND CAUSE OF
MASS POPULATION MOVEMENTS

Large populations can move rapidly in response to a single cataclysmic event (e.g., natural disaster) or a high-intensity political event (e.g., war). Populations can also move more gradually (seasonally or over years), such as migration toward urban or peri-urban areas for economic reasons or into new areas for agricultural reasons. Movement can be away from a bad situation, toward a promising one, or both (Prothero, 1989; Martens and Hall, 2000). Displaced populations can move into organized settings, such as planned refugee camps, into temporary or chaotic settings where minimal services are available, disperse into established communities, or remain highly mobile. The duration of dislocation or displacement can range from short (such as with seasonal work) to long-term or even permanent relocation. While returning a displaced population back home from a country or area of refuge is a fundamental goal, displacement can last for years or even decades, especially when its origins are political in nature. Displacement due to development projects, such as dams, can permanently alter the environment, making return impossible.

While this review focuses primarily on rapid movements of large populations and the recommendations provided are geared toward nongovernmental organizations (NGOs) providing humanitarian relief during such situations, the principles presented are derived primarily from malaria control in stable populations and could be applied to more slowly developing or more chronic situations.

The evolution of a complex humanitarian emergency (and, to some degree, any large, unplanned, rapid population movement) can be divided into two general phases: the emergency phase and the postemergency phase (Toole and Waldman, 1990).

Emergency Phase

The emergency phase of a complex emergency is often marked by increased mortality (exceeding 1 death per 10,000 population per day) (Bureau for Refugee Programs, 1985; Toole and Waldman, 1990; Centers for Disease Control, 1992; Burkholder and Toole, 1995; Meek et al., 1999). Priorities during this phase are directed toward addressing critical needs, such as provision of food, immunizations, water/sanitation, and shelter.

This phase may be characterized by outbreaks of communicable diseases, and health services often focus on case management for the most common illnesses and prevention of illnesses with the greatest epidemic potential.

A definition of the emergency phase was developed primarily to characterize a given situation and help prioritize public health interventions during emergencies occurring in developing countries where infectious diseases account for the bulk of morbidity and mortality. More recently, however, the nature of humanitarian crises in Kosovo and Bosnia-Herzegovina have brought into question the appropriateness of using mortality rates alone to define an emergency situation (Waldman and Martone, 1999; Spiegel and Salama, 2000, 2001; Waldman, 2001).

Postemergency Phase

The second stage is the postemergency or maintenance phase. During this period, the health profile of the displaced population returns to levels similar to preflight times and increasingly reflects the same communicable diseases that are present in the host population in the surrounding areas (Burkholder and Toole, 1995). It is during the postemergency phase that the focus of public health interventions for communicable diseases should shift from a predominantly curative approach to a sustainable, comprehensive approach that includes appropriate curative and prevention components, especially for common endemic diseases such as malaria. The goal of health care services during this period should be to maintain at acceptable levels, or further diminish, morbidity and mortality rates within the population.

POLITICAL AND ECONOMIC CAUSES OF
POPULATION MOVEMENT

War and severe political strife can disrupt health care services and disease control programs. Health care infrastructure can be destroyed or can simply cease to function. The food supply can be interrupted, causing deterioration in nutritional status. Homes and communities can be destroyed, and large populations may move in search of food, shelter, and safety.

A rapidly growing population can strain the capacity of rural areas and lead to population movement (Prothero, 1989; Martens and Hall, 2000). The search for new farmland causes people to encroach on forests and marginal lands. Large irrigation schemes are developed to produce food in arid areas. Dams are built, and roads are extended into remote areas. People who are no longer able to support themselves in rural areas move to urban areas in search of work or engage in such activities as logging, mining, and hunting that bring them into malaria-risk areas.

During the past 20 years, a large proportion of complex humanitarian emergencies have occurred in many regions where malaria is transmitted (see Figure 2-1). Many of the same socioeconomic forces that cause political instability also predispose areas to continued malaria transmission and vice versa. The drive for economic development can cause projects to be pushed forward with little or no consideration for health effects.

War and Civil Strife

In Southeast Asia, malaria was considered the primary cause of morbidity and mortality among Cambodian refugees when they first arrived in eastern Thailand in 1979 (Glass et al., 1980). Surveys conducted in Somalia during 1980 showed that, while malaria was not one of the leading causes of mortality, it still accounted for 2 to 5 percent of all deaths (Toole and Waldman, 1988). In 1984 among Karen refugees fleeing Myanmar to western Thailand, the annual incidence rate for malaria was 1,037 cases per thousand, with over 80 percent of infections due to *Plasmodium falciparum*, causing malaria control to be given high priority (Decludt et al., 1991). Malaria continues to be a major public health concern in these camps and surrounding areas (Brockman et al., 2000; Nosten et al., 2000; Chareonviriyaphap et al., 2000). In Central Asia, civil war and the attendant collapse of the health care infrastructure led to a reemergence of malaria in Tajikistan (Pitt et al., 1998). Recent relief efforts in East Timor and Afghanistan have been complicated by malaria (Ezard, 2001a; Sharp et al., 2002).

Similarly in Africa, malaria was the leading cause of death among adult Mozambican refugees in Malawi and among Ethiopian refugees in eastern Sudan (Centers for Disease Control, 1992). In the midst of massive cholera and dysentery epidemics at the beginning of the Rwandan refugee crisis in eastern Zaire (now the Democratic Republic of Congo) in 1994, fever presumed to be malaria was second only to diarrheal disease as the leading cause of morbidity and mortality (Goma Epidemiology Group, 1995; Centers for Disease Control and Prevention, 1996). In the years since the Rwandan refugee crisis, malaria has remained a major public health prob-

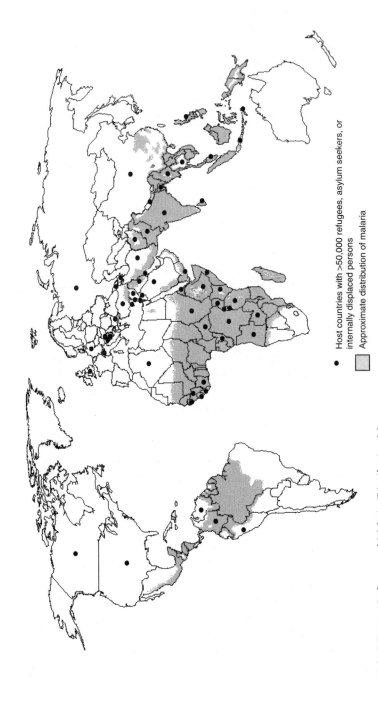

FIGURE 2-1   Refugees and Malaria: Distribution Map.
SOURCE: Adapted from U.S. Committee for Refugees (2000), World Health Organization (2002a), and Centers for Disease Control and Prevention (2000).

lem among displaced populations in the eastern Democratic Republic of Congo (International Rescue Committee, personal communications), Guinea (P. Spiegel, Centers for Disease Control and Prevention, personal communication, 2001; Ezard, 2001b) and Ethiopia (Salama et al., 2001).

Resettlement and Development

Resettlement typically refers to an organized relocation of large populations for purposes of population redistribution (e.g., "transmigration" in Indonesia), settlement of nomadic people, resettlement of repatriated refugees or demobilized military (Eritrea and Angola), social engineering (postcolonial Tanzania), or economic development (Brazil, Indonesia). Movement can be away from areas of development because of loss of land, such as occurs with dam building, or toward areas of development for purposes of employment (the latter is less likely to be an organized population movement).

The potential financial gains associated with economic development projects or large-scale commercial enterprises frequently attract large numbers of people. Often these movements are not organized and living conditions in new settlements can be poor, such as occurs with peri-urban slums or squatter's camps. The greater concentrations of people that occur can create highly focal areas of concern for malaria control, especially when the population is non-immune. In Brazil large groups of people travel from nonendemic areas into malarious areas to obtain work in mining operations and then become ill at very high rates (Veeken, 1993; de Andrade et al., 1995). Large-scale irrigation projects or hydroelectric water production schemes have been shown in many instances to facilitate mosquito breeding and malaria transmission (Kloos, 1990; Singh et al., 1999). In Indonesia, malaria has been identified as the primary public health concern of transmigrants and as a limitation to their acceptability of hydroelectric schemes (Abisudjak and Kotanegara, 1989).

Even relatively small-scale projects, such as road building or small dams, can have a large effect on malaria incidence through opening up malarious areas to travel (Hôpital le Bon Samaritain, Limbé, Haiti, unpublished surveillance data, 1965-1996), changing local environmental conditions, and attracting laborers (Sawyer, 1993; Alemayehu et al., 1998).

Urbanization

Between 1960 and 1980 the population living in urban settings in the developing world doubled (Knudsen and Sloof, 1992). This rapid urbanization of marginal areas within or on the outskirts of urban centers is commonly done in an uncontrolled fashion without thought or planning. Conditions are crowded; housing is of poor quality or of temporary construction; and the provision of health care, sanitation, and vectorborne disease control is inadequate. The result can be lack of proper drainage, leading to explosive growth of mosquito vectors, increased exposure to vectors due to poor housing, and amplification of disease to epidemic proportions through lack of effective treatment.

ENVIRONMENTAL AND NATURAL DISASTERS

Natural disasters, such as floods or earthquakes, can precipitate mass population movements out of affected areas or can cause a normally dispersed population to crowd around food and water sources, health care facilities, or debarkation points. Disasters involving flooding or severe rains can increase mosquito breeding sites (Mason and Cavalie, 1965). After a natural disaster a number of behavioral changes can occur that can increase the impact of malaria. Loss of housing or fear of collapsing structures can cause people to sleep outside, where contact with mosquitoes is increased. Normal health care services and disease control activities can be disrupted (Sáenz et al., 1995).

Hurricanes

Two to three months following a hurricane, Haiti experienced a severe epidemic of malaria that caused an estimated 75,000 cases (Mason and Cavalie, 1965). This epidemic was attributed to the presence of a considerable amount of malaria before the hurricane; destruction of shelter, putting people at increased risk of exposure; disruption of malaria control activities; massive increases in mosquito breeding sites due to rainfall and flooding; and a large influx of people to areas providing health care, food, and other assistance.

Earthquakes

After an earthquake in Costa Rica in 1991, malaria incidence increased between 1,600 and 4,700 percent in some affected cantons (Sáenz et al., 1995). These increases were associated with people being afraid to sleep indoors, disruption of malaria control activities in the area, and environmental changes due to the earthquake and flooding that allowed explosive growth in mosquito numbers.

Heavy Monsoon Rains/Floods

Heavy monsoon rains or other causes of flooding can dramatically increase mosquito breeding sites and result in massive increases in mosquito numbers. As with other natural disasters, heavy rains or flooding can disrupt normal malaria control efforts and destroy shelter, putting inhabitants at increased risk of acquiring malaria. Unusually heavy monsoon rains after the El Niño-Southern Oscillation (ENSO) in 1992 resulted in a malaria epidemic affecting four districts of Rajasthan, India, a typically arid region (Bouma and van der Kaay, 1994). Increased malaria transmission or epidemics have also occurred in association with ENSO events in Colombia, Uganda, Kenya, and elsewhere, although in the Tanzanian highlands malaria was reduced following the 1997-1998 ENSO (Bouma et al., 1997; Lindblade et al., 1999; Lindsay et al., 2000; Githeko et al., 2000).

Drought and Famine

Over the past 30 years, food shortages caused by drought and often exacerbated by war have been a frequent cause of population movements, especially in sub-Saharan Africa (Toole and Waldman, 1993; Prothero, 1994). In some cases, populations have been forced from malaria-free highland areas into endemic lowlands, exposing many of them to malaria for the first time and placing them at high risk of malaria-associated morbidity and mortality (Roundy, 1976; Mouchet et al., 1998; Anonymous, 1999).

**Speed, Duration, and Cause of
Mass Population Movements:
Key Points**

- Displacement can occur rapidly or slowly and can be caused by man-made (e.g., war, economic development) or naturally occurring situations (e.g., hurricanes, floods).

- Regardless of the cause of a complex emergency, there are generally two phases: emergency (focus on provision of curative health services) and postemergency (focus on prevention and sustainability).

- In addition to malaria having been a major public health threat for many displaced populations, human population movements in the past have resulted in the introduction or reintroduction of malaria into areas otherwise malaria free and the spread of anti-malarial drug resistance.

MALARIA-RELATED CHARACTERISTICS OF
MASS POPULATION MOVEMENTS

Large unplanned movements typically have a number of common attributes that increase not only people's risk of acquiring malaria but also the risk of epidemic malaria. Additionally, infrastructural changes or local and international politics may further complicate the provision of effective public health programs, exacerbating public health problems, including malaria.

Poor or No Housing

Studies conducted among stable populations living in malaria-endemic areas have shown that housing quality is associated with the risk of malaria infection (Koram et al., 1995a; Wolff et al., 2001). Similar problems have been noticed among refugee populations as well (Meek, 1989). Sub-standard shelter is common in situations where movement has been rapid and unplanned, such as occurs in refugee situations or when movement is expected to be temporary, such as movements for economic reasons. Substandard housing provides minimal or no protection from mosquitoes. Additionally, the areas in which people settle, whether refugee camps or peri-urban slums, are typically not planned with vector control in mind. Lack of planning for drainage of wastewater, for example, can create situations where explosive growth in vector populations is possible.

Movement into High-Risk Areas

Displaced populations are often forced to relocate or settle in areas with high risk of malaria. These can be areas that are unused by the stable population for specific reasons, such as known health risks (e.g., lack of safe water, known risk of disease). Migrant workers are often drawn to high-risk areas in search of work, such as mining in Brazil and Cambodia or logging in Myanmar and Thailand. Displaced populations may intentionally locate near water sources. While this facilitates the ready use of water, it may also put the population at increased risk of malaria if the water source is also a breeding site for mosquitoes.

Deliberate Movement to Areas Near Water

Displaced populations may intentionally locate near water sources. While this facilitates ready use of water, it may also put the population at increased risk of malaria if the water source is also a breeding site for mosquitoes.

Overcrowding

Crowding can increase the malaria burden among displaced populations by increasing the density and proximity of both infected individuals and susceptible people. This phenomenon is seen even among stable populations exposed to fairly constant levels of transmission (Defo, 1995).

Low Socioeconomic Status

Within stable populations, low socioeconomic status has been associated with increased risk of malaria (Koram et al., 1995a). The exact reason for this is unclear, but it may be related to decreased access to health care, limited knowledge of risk factors, poor housing, marginal nutritional status, or behaviors that put individuals at increased risk of malaria.

Proximity of Livestock

A number of explanations have been offered for a reported two-fold higher prevalence of malaria among Afghan refugees living in Pakistan, as compared with local Pakistani residents. One is that the refugees came from an area of low malaria endemicity to an area of higher endemicity and were at increased risk because of low population-level immunity (Suleman, 1988). Other explanations focus on "zooprophylaxis" (Service, 1990). Some malaria vector mosquitoes will feed preferentially on livestock if available; if insufficient numbers of livestock are kept nearby, mosquitoes may begin to feed on humans. Conversely, livestock may attract mosquitoes, which may feed on nearby people if the opportunity arises, causing increased exposure to malaria (Hewitt et al., 1994; Bouma and Rowland, 1995; Mouchet et al., 1998). Information on the behavior of the specific vectors in the area is essential to understand the potential impact of livestock on malaria risk.

Mobility

Movement back and forth between settlement areas and areas of high malaria risk ("circulation") can increase people's exposure to malaria and the risk of introduction of the disease into malaria-free areas (Prothero, 1977). In Thailand a well-described cause of epidemic malaria is the movement of people between the forested areas of the Thai-Myanmar and Thai-Cambodian borders, where malaria risk is high, and nonendemic low-land villages. Most of the movement is for economic reasons, including logging, hunting, and charcoal making (Singhanetra-Renard, 1993; Chareonviriyaphap et al., 2000).

Immune Status

Understanding the interaction between the probable immune status of populations in transition and the intensity of malaria transmission to which they will be exposed is exceedingly important in anticipating the likely impact of malaria.

Displaced populations can move from an area of high malaria transmission to another area of high transmission. Although there are some indications that, because of antigenic or strain variation, an adequate or protective immune response in one area does not guarantee an adequate or protective immune response in another area, typically this situation carries the least risk in terms of increased morbidity or mortality. Population-level immunity would be expected to be high and, while malaria may still be a major cause of illness and death, it would not be expected to be clinically worse than it would be in the area of origin.

A far more serious situation occurs when displaced populations from an area of low or no malaria risk arrive in an area with high transmission. Because the overall level of immunity would be low, a significant risk of severe illness and death exists. In these situations an aggressive malaria control program becomes essential; not only is ready access to effective curative services needed, preventive measures, including comprehensive public education, should be included.

A similar level of concern should be given to addressing malaria risk among nonimmune responders (see Chapter 10, Prophylaxis and Personal Protection for Aid Workers). Relief workers and other personnel responding to displacement situations are frequently from nonendemic areas and can be at high risk of malaria-associated morbidity and mortality. For example, U.N. Peacekeepers in the Democratic Republic of Congo and Sierra Leone have reportedly had a serious problem with malaria, resulting in increased sick-leave and even deaths (C. Halle, U.N. Department of Peacekeeping Operations, personal communication, 2002).

Finally, displaced populations can move from an area of high transmission to an area of low or no malaria risk. Many areas, countries, or regions have successfully eradicated malaria even though competent mosquito vectors still exist. In this situation, concern should include not only treatment of clinical cases as they occur but also reduction of the likelihood of introduction or reintroduction of malaria. Strategies to accomplish this include screening or presumptive therapy of new arrivals and vector control. Because immunity to malaria wanes over time in the absence of exposure, displaced populations spending as little as one or two years away from their homes in endemic regions should be considered nonimmune and appropriate precautions should be instituted upon repatriation or resettlement to malaria-endemic areas.

A similar problem exists if the areas of origin and refuge differ with regard to the prevalence of drug-resistant malaria. Refugees arriving in an area where little or no drug resistance occurs from another area where drug-resistant malaria is common can act as a source of introduction of resistance. This can be an issue both with newly arriving refugees and with repatriation back to the country of origin.

It is possible that new arrivals will come with different histories of previous exposure. Rwandan refugees arriving in the Democratic Republic of Congo (then Zaire) in 1994, for example, came from all over Rwanda, including some highland areas where malaria risk is lower or nonexistent. The prevailing treatment policy at the time, however, was use of chloroquine, despite high levels of resistance to that drug. While an individual with acquired immunity can still respond adequately to a marginally effective antimalarial drug, one who comes from an area with little or no malaria transmission (and therefore little or no acquired immunity) would likely be at risk of severe complications or even death.

While an individual's level of acquired immunity can affect the clinical presentation of malaria (see Chapter 3, section on Epidemiology of Clinical Malaria), malaria infection can increase the risk of infection or modify the progression of disease due to other pathogens, through either direct immunosuppression or other alterations in host factors. Evidence of such interactions exists for *Salmonella* and human immunodeficiency virus and may also exist for tuberculosis (Mabey et al., 1987; Xiao et al., 1998; Hoffman et al., 1999; Enwere et al., 1999). Malaria infection can reduce the immune response to vaccines for tetanus, typhoid, and meningitis (Greenwood et al., 1981). Successful prevention of malaria through combined use of insecticide-impregnated bed nets and chemoprophylaxis resulted in a significant drop in mortality from all causes among Gambian children, suggesting a substantial indirect effect on nonmalarial illness (Alonso et al., 1993).

Nutritional Deficiency

The interaction between malnutrition and malaria is complex and not well understood. Studies of the interaction between nutrition and malaria have had conflicting results (Hendrikse et al., 1971; Murray et al., 1977; Oppenheimer et al., 1986a; Greenwood et al., 1987; Smith et al., 1989; Snow et al., 1991; van Hensbroek et al., 1995). A critical evaluation of these studies, their methodologies, and their interpretations, though, suggests that protein energy malnutrition is in fact associated with an increase in malaria morbidity and mortality (Shankar, 2000). Information collected during famine relief efforts suggests that nutritional rehabilitation of famine victims can induce recrudescence of sequestered parasites, causing an increase in malaria, and that refeeding programs should include provisions for malaria prevention (Murray et al., 1976, 1978; Shankar, 2000).

The effects of specific micronutrient deficiencies on malaria morbidity and mortality is equally complex and requires more investigation. The effect of specific micronutrient deficiencies may be reflected not only in greater susceptibility to malaria (e.g., increased incidence or higher parasite densities) but also poorer response to malaria therapy. For example, the prevalence and degree of parasitological resistance to both chloroquine and sulfadoxine/pyrimethamine were worse among malnourished Rwandan refugees, possibly because of impairment of immune function (Wolday et al., 1995).

While malaria may be exacerbated by certain nutritional deficiencies, malnutrition can also be worsened because of it. Malaria causes increased red blood cell destruction and decreased production, further complicating preexisting nutritional anemias (Greenwood, 1987). The anorexia and vomiting frequently associated with malaria infection can limit food intake (McGregor, 1982). One study even raised the question of whether *P. vivax* infection might be a cause of acute malnutrition in Vanuatu (Williams et al., 1997).

Destruction or Overburdening of Existing Infrastructure

In many settings, local health care infrastructure may be lacking or inadequate to deal with a large, newly arrived population. After natural disasters and war, disruption of normally adequate infrastructure can occur. There may be insufficient numbers of buildings, equipment, and trained staff. Drugs and medical supplies may be inadequate and difficult to obtain. Normal disease control efforts can also be disrupted, contributing to epidemics, as occurred in Costa Rica after an earthquake (Sáenz et al., 1995).

The logistics of supplying and supporting services may also change dramatically. Roads may become impassable. The population may move to remote areas where existing services or roads are inadequate for large-scale movement of supplies. Trucks and other vehicles, spare parts, trained mechanics, and fuel may all be in short supply.

Availability of Health Care

Although governments and international agencies go to great lengths to provide health care services in emergency situations, it is not always apparent to the population being served where or how to access that care. The availability of health care services must also be sufficient for the size of the population. Surveys conducted in refugee camps in Goma, Zaire, found that 47 percent of people dying from diarrheal disease had never visited a health care facility (Goma Epidemiology Group, 1995). Overall, more than 90 percent of deaths from all causes occurred outside health care facilities, suggesting that health care services were not accessible to most of the population or that the demand for curative services overwhelmed the capacity of the organizations (Centers for Disease Control and Prevention, 1996). A malaria control strategy based on prompt, effective therapy of acute febrile illness can only be successful if people know where to go to get diagnosed and treated and if such facilities are easily accessible.

Operational Concerns

Nongovernmental organizations frequently suffer from high turnover of staff, causing a loss of institutional knowledge. Expatriate staff often lack specialized knowledge or experience with tropical diseases, especially malaria.

Coordination of malaria control efforts across organizations can be an impediment to successful implementation of malaria control activities. Often, there is no clearly identified lead agency responsible for coordinating the implementation of these activities. Responsibilities related to malaria control may be divided between nongovernmental organizations and other multinational organizations: one may be responsible for curative health care, another for environmental control, still another for outreach or other community-based interventions. Unfortunately, these various agencies work under different and, at times, conflicting paradigms and agendas.

Donor Fatigue

As complex emergencies or other situations involving mass population movements become prolonged affairs, international support can wane. International relief organizations move on to the next emergency. Some transfer responsibility to local nongovernmental organizations that may not have the international visibility needed to supplement diminishing public financial support. Responsibility may also shift to the government of the host country, which may already be hard pressed to provide adequate services to its own citizens. Additionally, high-cost interventions may be introduced by comparatively well-funded international agencies that the inheriting local nongovernmental organization or government might have a difficult time sustaining. Examples include the first-line use of relatively expensive antimalarial drugs or rapid diagnostic ("dipstick") methods that are not a normal part of the host country's national formulary or practices.

Factors Affecting Overall Risk of Malaria: Key Points

- Large, unplanned movements can increase both the risk of acquiring malaria and the risk of epidemics.

- Factors influencing the overall risk of malaria include poor or no housing, movement into unused areas, deliberate movement to areas near water, overcrowding, low socioeconomic status, proximity of livestock, mobility, immune status, and under- and malnutrition.

- Political and infrastructural factors that affect the provision of health care services include destruction or overburdening of existing infrastructure, limited availability of health care services, insufficient or poorly trained staff, insufficient coordination among agencies, and donor fatigue.

- Most of the above factors operate simultaneously in a complex emergency and must be considered when planning realistic malaria control strategies.

3

Epidemiology of Malaria

A familiarity with the technical aspects of malaria is necessary for decisions to be made about how to devise a locally appropriate malaria control strategy. Such familiarity can aid in determining whether malaria might pose an important public health risk in a given situation, how large a problem it might be, which drugs would be expected to be effective and which probably would not, and which groups within a displaced population might be at increased risk of malaria and therefore need special attention.

The following section presents information on areas at risk of malaria transmission, the mechanics of how malaria is transmitted within a population, the range of clinical manifestations of malaria, antimalarial drug resistance, and the mosquito vector. The information presented is by no means exhaustive but should aid in basic decision making or in recognizing when expert assistance is needed.

AREAS AT RISK

Malaria occurs primarily in tropical and some subtropical regions of Africa, Central and South America, Asia, and Oceania (Figure 2-1). In areas where malaria occurs, there is tremendous variation in the intensity of transmission and risk of infection. For example, over 90 percent of clinical malaria infections and deaths occur in sub-Saharan Africa (World Health Organization, 1996a). However, even there the risk varies widely. Highland (>1,500 m) and arid areas (<1,000 mm rainfall/year) typically have less malaria, although these areas are prone to epidemic malaria if climactic conditions become favorable to mosquito development (World Health Organization, 1996a). Although urban areas have typically been at lower risk, explosive unplanned population growth has been a major factor in making urban or peri-urban transmission an increasing problem (Knudsen and Sloof, 1992).

Human malaria is caused by one or more of four parasites: *Plasmodium falciparum*, *P. vivax*, *P. ovale*, and *P. malariae*. Distribution of these parasites varies geographically, and not all species of malaria are transmitted in all malarious areas. *P. falciparum*, the species most commonly associated with fatal malaria, is transmitted at some level in nearly all areas where malaria occurs. It accounts for over 90 percent of all malaria infections in sub-Saharan Africa, for nearly 100 percent of infections in Haiti, and causes two-thirds or more of the malaria cases in Southeast Asia. *P. vivax* is a relatively uncommon infection in sub-Saharan Africa. Duffy antigens, which are required by the parasite to invade red blood cells, are lacking in many ethnic groups, especially in West Africa. Vivax malaria, however, is the predominant species in Central America, most of malarious South America, and the Indian subcontinent (Miller et al., 1977).

MECHANISMS OF INFECTION AND TRANSMISSION

Malaria is typically transmitted by the bite of an infective female *Anopheles* mosquito; transmission can also occur transplacentally, as a result of blood transfusion, or by needle sharing. Infective mosquitoes inject sporozoites into the bloodstream during feeding (see Figure 3-1). These sporozoites infect liver cells (b) where they undergo asexual reproduction (exoerythrocytic schizogony), producing schizonts (c). In 6 to 14 days (sometimes longer), the schizonts rupture, releasing merozoites into the bloodstream (d). Merozoites invade red blood cells and undergo a second phase of asexual reproduction (erythrocytic schizogony), developing into rings (e), trophozoites (f), and finally blood stage schizonts (g). The schizonts rupture, destroying the red blood cell and releasing more merozoites into the bloodstream, starting another cycle of asexual development and multiplication (h). This erythocytic cycle will continue until the infected individual is successfully treated, mounts an immune response that clears the infection, or dies. During this cycle, sexual forms called gametocytes are produced (i) and can be ingested by a mosquito during a

26

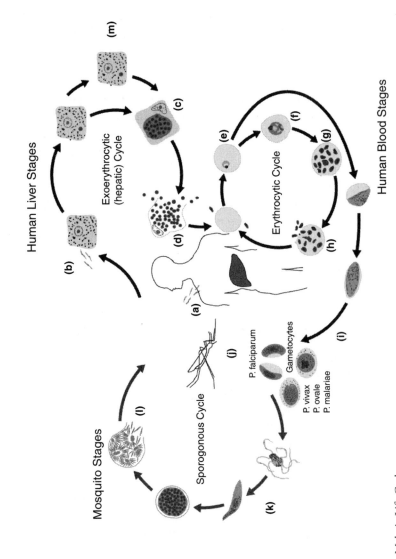

FIGURE 3-1 Malaria Life Cycle.

blood meal (j). Sexual reproduction occurs in the mosquito (k). Sporozoites are formed (l), which migrate to the salivary glands, making the mosquito infective to humans.

The timing of events in the life cycle of malaria parasites and the number of merozoites produced during schizogony vary by species. Additionally, two species of malaria, *P. vivax* and *P. ovale*, have a form, "hypnozoites" (m), that can persist in the liver for months to years, causing periodic relapses of peripheral parasitemia and illness (see Table 3-1).

MALARIA VECTORS AND VECTOR BEHAVIOR

Human malaria is transmitted by the bite of female mosquitoes belonging to the genus *Anopheles*. Of the 400 or so species of *Anopheles* in the world, approximately 60 are important vectors of malaria. However, a particular species of *Anopheles* may be an important vector in one area of the world and of little or no consequence in another.

Different species of *Anopheles* can behave differently. Mosquito behavior can differ in terms of breeding or larval habitat (e.g., fresh vs. brackish water; flowing streams, still pools, or man-made habitats; shaded or sunny sites), feeding preferences (e.g., time of day when peak biting occurs, preferences for people over animals, feeding indoors or outside), and resting habits (resting indoors after feeding or leaving the house before resting). These differences in mosquito behavior can affect both the epidemiology of malaria and the choice of malaria control strategy used. For example, *An. dirus* is an important vector in Southeast Asia and is primarily a forest dweller. People at greatest risk are, therefore, those who enter the forest for whatever reason, while those who stay closer to home (such as small children) are at less risk. This also means that malaria control strategies aimed at preventing mosquito biting in the home (such as residual spraying or insecticide-treated bed nets) would be of little value in preventing exposure and infection. *An. gambiae,* the most important vector in much of sub-Saharan Africa, breed in small temporary pools of water (even as small and temporary as cattle hoofprints). Therefore, vector control strategies aimed at reducing or eliminating breeding sites will likely have little impact. For these reasons, expert advice relevant to the primary malaria vectors in a given area is essential for making sound decisions regarding control options.

TABLE 3-1 Characteristics of the Four Species of Human Malaria

	P. falciparum	*P. vivax*	*P. ovale*	*P. malariae*
Exoerythrocytic cycle	6-7 Days	6-8 Days	9 Days	14-16 Days
Prepatent period	9-10 Days	11-13 Days	10-14 Days	15-16 Days
Incubation period (mean)	9-14 (12) Days	12-17 (15) Days to 6-12 months	16-18 (17) Days or longer	18-40 (28) Days or longer
Severity of primary attack	Severe	Mild to severe	Severe	Severe
Duration of primary attack[a]	16-36 Hours or longer	8-12 Hours	8-12 Hours	8-10 Hours
Duration of untreated infection[a]	1-2 Years	1.5-5 Years	1.5-5 Years	3-50 Years
Relapse	No	Yes	Yes	No
Central nervous system complications[a]	Frequent	Infrequent	Infrequent	Infrequent
Anemia[a]	Frequent	Common	Infrequent	Infrequent
Renal insufficiency[a]	Common	Infrequent	Infrequent	Infrequent
Effects on pregnancy[a]	Frequent	Infrequent	Unknown	Unknown
Hypoglycemia	Frequent	Unknown	Unknown	Unknown

[a] Influenced by immunity. Documentation of complications for species other than *P. falciparum* is limited.
SOURCE: Adapted from Bruce-Chwatt (1985).

VECTOR LIFE CYCLE

There are four stages in the life cycle of the mosquito: egg, larva, pupa, and adult. Eggs are deposited singly on water in suitable breeding sites, where the developing embryo hatches as a larva after 2 or more days. During the aquatic period of development, the larva sheds its skin four times. The fourth larval molt gives rise to a pupa. At this stage the mosquito undergoes a complete metamorphosis, emerging as an adult. When parasites are ingested during a blood meal, they undergo further development in the mosquito's stomach, and during the next 10 to 20 days the parasite passes through a number of stages, eventually multiplying and penetrating all parts of the mosquito body. Parasites that end up in the salivary glands can be transmitted to humans when the mosquito takes another blood meal.

The length of each developmental stage depends on temperature and humidity. The life span of adults under natural conditions is difficult to determine but averages 10 to 14 days or longer (Service, 1993). The time for an egg to develop to an adult in the tropics can be as short as 5 to 7 days. Development of malaria parasites in the mosquito host is also temperature dependent; as ambient temperatures decrease, the time needed for parasites to develop increases. Malaria transmission stops when the time needed for development of infective sporozoites exceeds the life span of the mosquito (Gilles, 1993).

MALARIA ILLNESS

The normal incubation period from infective mosquito bite to onset of clinical symptoms is 9 to 30 days or longer, depending on such parameters as species of parasite, immune status, infecting dose, and use of antimalarial drugs. The clinical symptoms associated with malaria parasites are produced by increases in cytokines (particularly tumor necrosis factor) in response to merozoites, pyrogens, and cellular debris released when red blood cells rupture at the end of schizogony (Kwiatkowski, 1990). Onset of illness is associated with the initial rupture of erythrocytic schizonts; exoerythrocytic forms (sporozoites, exoerythrocytic schizonts, and hypnozoites) and gametocytes do not cause clinical symptoms.

Typical symptoms among nonimmune individuals include fever, chills, myalgias and arthralgias, headache, diarrhea, and other nonspecific signs. Other findings may include splenomegaly, anemia, thrombocytopenia, pulmonary or renal dysfunction, changes in mental status, and coma. Most cases of malaria-related severe illness and death are associated with *P. falciparum* infection. This is due, in part, to the parasite's ability to infect both mature and immature red blood cells, its rapid rate of asexual reproduction, and a broad range of poorly understood pathological processes associated with its ability to sequester in postcapillary venules, especially in the central nervous system. Cyclical fevers seen in nonimmune individuals with synchronous infections (occurring when a majority of schizonts rupture at the same time) are frequently absent among individuals with immunity.

In general, immunity to malaria is acquired after repeated exposure to the malaria parasite; those individuals who survive their initial infections develop some degree of immunity. In highly endemic areas, most clinical malaria and malaria-associated mortality occurs in children less than 5 years old, whose immunity has not yet fully developed. Although malaria prevalence in endemic areas decreases with increasing age, suggesting an acquired ability to clear malaria infections, immunity to malaria typically also involves the development of a tolerance for the presence of malaria parasites in the blood with a minimum of symptoms and relative protection from severe illness and death.

EPIDEMIOLOGY OF CLINICAL MALARIA

Malaria transmission intensity, levels of acquired immunity in a population, and manifestations of malaria illness are intimately linked (see Table 3-2; Snow et al., 1994; Slutsker et al., 1994). Understanding this relationship should help in estimating the likely impact of malaria in a given population. An important additional consideration is understanding the implications of differences between the environment from which a displaced population comes and the environment in which that population settles, even if only temporarily.

The overall level of immunity to malaria is highest in areas where malaria transmission is the most intense. The first exposure to malaria occurs very early in childhood, and with repeated exposures the likelihood of severe illness or death lessens. In Africa, where the majority of malaria-associated deaths occur, the highest mortality rates occur in children less than 5 years old. It has been estimated that in the Gambia, malaria accounts for 25 percent of all deaths among children less than 5 years old. Malaria-associated mortality decreases rapidly with increasing age (Greenwood et

TABLE 3-2 Malaria Transmission Characteristics, Immunity, and Clinical Features

Areas Where *P. falciparum* Malaria Is Predominant or Represents a Significant Proportion of Infecting Malaria Species			Areas Where Nonfalciparum Malaria Is the Predominant Infecting Species
Areas of Intense Perennial Malaria Transmission and/or Populations with High Levels of Immunity Originating in Those Areas	Areas of Low-to-Moderate Malaria Transmission	Areas of Very Low, Highly Seasonal, or Epidemic Malaria Transmission and/or Low Levels of Immunity in the Population	*Examples:* Central America, some parts of the Indian subcontinent, parts of Central Asia, parts of eastern Europe. *Typical epidemiology of clinical illness:*
Example: Most of tropical equatorial Africa. *Typical epidemiology of clinical illness:* Bulk of clinical disease occurs in young (<5 years old) children. While adults and older children are often parasitemic, they are more likely to be asymptomatically infected or to have only mild symptoms. Severe anemia tends to be more common than cerebral malaria in young children.	*Examples:* Parts of southern Africa, coastal eastern Africa, Indian subcontinent, Southeast Asia. *Typical epidemiology of clinical illness:* Bulk of disease occurs in broader range of ages. Cerebral malaria becomes more common.	*Examples:* Sahelian and highland areas of Africa, Central America. *Typical epidemiology of clinical illness:* Disease can occur in all age groups and is more likely to progress to severe disease if not promptly treated. In some areas of very low transmission (e.g., Haiti), mortality rates associated with malaria can be paradoxically low, probably due to high incidence of clinical symptoms, rapid treatment-seeking behavior of the population, and the high efficacy and ready availability of CQ.	Nonfalciparum malaria can be a significant cause of morbidity but is rarely associated with severe illness or death. Spontaneous splenic rupture can occur in chronic *P. vivax* infections, but cerebral malaria has only rarely been attributed to this parasite. Infections caused by *P. malariae* have been associated with nephrotic syndrome. In areas where both falciparum and nonfalciparum malaria occur, species-specific treatment is advisable. Because drugs used for the treatment of acute infections do not typically affect the hypnozoites of *P. ovale* and *P. vivax*, these infections can relapse months to years later.

al., 1987; Campbell, 1991). In areas with very high levels of transmission, severe malaria tends to manifest itself more frequently as anemia than as cerebral disease. As transmission intensity decreases and population immunity is lessened, illness is seen more frequently in all age groups and the incidence of cerebral disease increases relative to severe anemia.

Displaced populations coming from areas of little or no malaria transmission to areas with intense transmission are therefore at greatest risk of severe illness and death due to a lack of acquired immunity. Until they themselves acquire a protective level of immunity to malaria, these populations will probably require a much more intensive intervention effort to achieve and maintain low rates of morbidity and mortality.

Malaria also has important effects in the way of chronic or repeated infections, including anemia (especially among individuals with underlying malnutrition), and poor pregnancy outcomes. Anemia, itself an important cause of mortality associated with malaria, is also a common reason for blood transfusion.

MALARIA DURING PREGNANCY

Among nonimmune women, acute malaria during pregnancy carries a high risk of maternal and fetal death if not treated promptly and adequately. Among semiimmune pregnant women, however, malaria parasites preferentially sequester in the placenta, with minimal increase in overt clinical disease. Malaria during pregnancy is a cause of both maternal anemia and low birth weight, accounting for as much as 35 percent of preventable low birth weight in malarious areas (Steketee et al., 1996a). Low birth weight, in turn, is a well-recognized risk factor for infant mortality (McCormick, 1985). In most populations living in areas of high malaria transmission, this is an issue primarily affecting women in their first and second pregnancies.

MALARIA AND HIV/AIDS

Malaria and HIV infection can occur at high frequencies in the same population, especially in sub-Saharan Africa, raising concerns that interactions between these two diseases could greatly complicate control of both (Corbett et al., 2002). Malaria and HIV have indeed been shown to interact in important ways. Peripheral malaria infection has been shown to occur more frequently and parasite densities have been shown to be higher among HIV-positive pregnant women compared with HIV-negative pregnant women (Steketee et al., 1996b). HIV-infected women are at increased risk of placental malaria, even during later pregnancies when placental sequestration is less of a problem among HIV-negative women (Steketee et al., 1996b). Similarly, HIV-infected, nonpregnant individuals are at increased risk of both malaria infection and illness (Whitworth et al., 2000). There is also evidence that acute malaria infection can increase viral load among HIV-infected individuals, an increase that is reversed with effective malaria therapy (Hoffman et al., 1999). Finally, unscreened blood transfusions for malaria-associated anemia remain an important source of HIV transmission in malarious areas (Corbett, et al., 2002).

ANTIMALARIAL DRUG RESISTANCE

Simply defined, antimalarial drug resistance occurs when malaria parasites gain the ability to survive what should be an effective dose of antimalarial drugs. Resistance occurs because of naturally occurring mutations that affect the susceptibility of the parasite to a given drug. For some drugs, resistance can occur after a single-point mutation (as for the drug atovaquone); with others a number of mutations may be required. Factors that facilitate intensification of drug resistance include poor adherence to recommended treatment regimens, inadequate dosing, use of poor-quality drugs, presumptive treatment, and use of drugs that have a long half-life. Because of rapidly developing and spreading resistance to antimalarials and the relatively slow process of developing new antimalarials, the number of useful drugs is dwindling (Bloland and Ettling, 1999; Winstanley, 2000). The most commonly available antimalarial drugs are described in Appendix A and Table 3-3, although not all are practical or appropriate for use in any given situation.

Chloroquine-resistant *P. falciparum* (CRPF) was first recognized almost simultaneously in Thailand and South America in the late 1950s. It was first identified on the east coast of Africa in 1978. In the past 20 to 25 years, CRPF has spread and intensified to the point that only Central America northwest of the Panama Canal, the island of Hispaniola (Haiti and the Dominican Republic), and limited regions of the Middle East are free of chloroquine (CQ) resistance. All other endemic areas have malaria that is, to varying extents, resistant to CQ. In some regions, CQ resistance has intensified to the point where the drug no longer has an optimal effect

TABLE 3-3 Antimalarial Drugs for Uncomplicated Malaria

Combination Therapy

| Drug Name | Use | Dosing (all per os)[a] | | Contra-indications | Cost (US$)[b] | Comments |
		Adult	Pediatric			
MQ + artesunate	Treatment of nonsevere falciparum infections thought to be CQ and SP-resistant.	15 mg/kg MQ base on day 2 of treatment, followed by 10 mg/kg MQ base on day 3. Usual adult dose is 750 mg on day 2 followed by 500 mg on day 3.	15 mg/kg MQ on day 2 of treatment followed by 10 mg/kg MQ on day 3.	See under MQ monotherapy.	3.90	Safety of artemisinins and MQ during first trimester of pregnancy not established. Vomiting after MQ can be reduced by administering it on the second and third days after an initial dose of artesunate. Artemisinin (20 mg/kg initially followed by 10 mg/kg once daily for 2 more days) can be substituted can besubstituted for artesunate.
		4 mg/kg artesunate daily for 3 days.	4 mg/kg artesunate daily for 3 days.			

Drug	Indication	Dosing	Dosing	Contraindications		Comments
SP + artesunate	Treatment of nonsevere falicparum infections thought to be CQ resistant.	As for SP monotherapy (see below).	As for SP monotherapy (see below).	Known SP allergy.	1.12	This combination has not been evaluated as extensively as MQ + artesunate. Safety of artemisinin during first trimester of pregnancy not established. Artemisinin (as described above) can be substituted for artesunate.
		4 mg/kg artesunate daily for 3 days.	4 mg/kg artesunate daily for 3 days.			
CQ or amodiaquine + artesunate	Treatment of CQ-resistant malaria.	Treatment: 25 mg base/kg divided over 3 days.	Treatment: 25 mg base/kg divided over 3 days.			Combination of amodiaquine + artesunate generally more useful due to widespread, typically high-level CQ resistance. In some areas,

continued

TABLE 3-3 Continued

Drug Name	Use	Dosing (all per os)[a]		Contra-indications	Cost (US$)[b]	Comments
		Adult	Pediatric			
		Average adult dose: 2.5 gm (salt) divided over 3 days.				neither would be expected to be particularly effective.
		4 mg/kg artesunate daily for 3 days.	4 mg/kg artesunate daily for 3 days.			See note below on possible toxicity associated with amodiaquine.
Lumefantrine/ artemether also known as: co-aremether Trade names: Coartem, Riamet	Treatment of multidrug-resistant malaria.	Adult: 4 tablets per dose at 0, 8, 24, 36, 48, and 60 hours.	Pediatric: 10-14 kg: 1 tablet/dose 15-24 kg: 2 tablets/dose 25-35 kg: 3 tablets/dose >35 kg: as for adult given at 0, 8, 24, 36, 48, and 60 hours.	Hypersensitivity to component drugs.	2.40 (WHO price only)	Commercially available fixed-dose combination of 20 mg artemether and 120 mg lumefantrine. Not recommended for <10 kg or pregnant women Available in 2 packaging schemes: 24 tablet/6 doses (Riamet) and 16 tablets/

CQ (or amodiaquine) + sulfadoxine/ pyrimethamine	Treatment of CQ-resistant malaria.	Use routine doses for both CQ/ amodiaquine and SP.	Use routine doses for both CQ/ amodiaquine and SP.	Same as for CQ/ amodiaquine and SP monotherapy.	4 doses. (Coartem)— 4 dose regimen not as effective especially for nonimmunes. Also available from WHO in specially designed blister packs. Primarily useful only in areas where CQ resistance is low to moderate and SP resistance is low. See notes of caution regarding use of amodiaquine.

Single-Agent Therapy

CQ Trade names: Nivaquine, Malaraquine, Aralen, many others	Treatment of nonfalciparum infections. Treatment of P. falciparum infections in areas where CQ remains effective.	Treatment: 25 mg base/kg divided over 3 days. Average adult: 1.5 gm base divided over	Treatment: 25 mg base/kg divided over 3 days.	0.08	Widespread resistance in P. falciparum in most regions. Resistance in P. vivax occurs in some areas. Can cause pruritus in dark-skinned patients, reducing compliance.

continued

TABLE 3-3 Continued

Drug Name	Use	Dosing (all per os)[a] Adult	Pediatric	Contra-indications	Cost (US$)[b]	Comments
	Chemoprophylaxis in areas where CQ remains effective.	3 days. Prophylaxis: 5 mg/kg base per week.	Prophylaxis: 5 mg base/kg once per week.			Preparations differ in amount of base (100 or 150 mg tablets, 50 mg syrup).
Amodiaquine Trade names: Camoquine, others	Treatment of nonsevere falicparum infections thought to be CQ resistant.	Treatment: 25 mg base/kg divided over 3 days. Single dose of 25 mg (sulfa)/kg	Treatment: 25 mg base/kg divided over 3 days. Single dose of 25 mg (sulfa)/kg		0.14	Cross-resistance with CQ limits usefulness in areas with high rates of CQ resistance. Has been associated with toxic hepatitis and agranulocytosis when used as prophylaxis; risk when used for treatment unknown.
SP Trade name: Fansidar, others	Treatment of nonsevere falicparum infections thought to be CQ resistant.	Average adult: 3 tablets as a single dose.	By age: • <1 year, 1/2 tablet • 1-2 years, 3/4 tablet • 3-5 years, 1 tablet	Known sulfa allergy.	0.12	Efficacy for vivax infections may be poor. Widespread resistance in P. falciparum in some regions.

Sulfalene/ pyrimethamine (Metakelfin)		• 6-8 years, 1.5 tablets • 9-11 years, 2 tablets • 12-13 years, 2.5 tablets • >14 years, 3 tablets			Can cause severe skin disease when used prophylactically; risk when used as treatment unknown but likely to be very low.
MQ Trade names: Larium, Mephaquine	Treatment of nonsevere falicparum infections thought to be CQ and SP resistant. Chemoprophylaxis in areas with CQ resistance.	Treatment: 750 to 1,500 mg base depending on local resistance patterns. Larger doses (>15 mg/kg) best given in split doses over 2 days. Prophylaxis: 250 mg once per week.	Treatment: 15-25 mg base/kg depending on local resistance patterns. Larger doses (>15 mg/kg) best given in split doses over 2 days. Prophylaxis: 5 mg base/kg once per week.	Known or suspected history of neuro-psychiatric disorder, history of seizures, concomitant use of halofantrine.	1.92	Vomiting can be a common problem in young children. In some populations (e.g., very young African children), unpredictable blood levels, even after appropriate dosing, can produce frequent treatment failure.

continued

TABLE 3-3 Continued

Drug Name	Use	Dosing (all per os)[a]		Contra-indications	Cost (US$)[b]	Comments
		Adult	Pediatric			
Halofantrine Trade name: Halfan	Treatment of suspected multidrug-resistant falciparum.	8 mg base/kg every 6 hours for 3 doses. Average adult: 1,500 mg base divided into 3 doses as above.	8 mg base/kg every 6 hours for 3 doses.	Preexisting cardiac disease, congenital prolongation of QT_c interval, treatment with MQ within prior 3 weeks, pregnancy.	5.31	Cross-resistance with MQ has been reported. Reported to have highly variable bioavailability. Risk of fatal cardiotoxicity.
Quinine	Treatment of severe malaria. Treatment of multidrug-resistant P. falciparum. Treatment of malaria	Nonsevere malaria: 8 mg base/kg 3 times daily for 7 days.	Nonsevere malaria: 8 mg base/kg 3 times daily for 7 days.		1.51	Side effects can greatly reduce compliance. Used in combination with tetracycline, doxycycline, clindamycin, or SP (where effective) and in areas where

Drug		Average adult dose	Child dose	Contraindications		Comments
	during first trimester of pregnancy.	Average adult: 650 mg 3 times daily for 7 days. Severe: see section on treatment of severe malaria.	Severe: see section on treatment of severe malaria.			quinine resistance is not prevalent, duration of quinine dosage can be reduced to 3 days.
Tetracycline (tetra)/ doxycycline (doxy)	In combination with quinine, can increase efficacy of treatment in areas with quinine resistance and/or reduce likelihood of quinine-associated side effects by reducing duration of quinine treatment. Prophylaxis.	Tetra: 250 mg/ 4 times per day for 7 days. Doxy: 100 mg 2 times per day for 7 days. Prophylaxis: 100 mg doxy per day.	Tetra: 5 mg/kg 4 times per day for 7 days. Doxy: 2 mg/kg twice per day for 7 days. Prophylaxis: 2mg/kg doxy per day up to 100 mg.	Age less than 8 years, pregnancy.	0.14- 0.20	Used only in combination with a rapidly acting schizonticide such as quinine.

continued

TABLE 3-3 Continued

Drug Name	Use	Dosing (all per os)[a]		Contra-indications	Cost (US$)[b]	Comments
		Adult	Pediatric			
Clindamycin	For patients unable to take tetracycline. In combination with quinine, can increase efficacy of treatment in areas with quinine resistance and/or reduce likelihood of quinine-associated side effects by reducing duration of quinine treatment.	300 mg 4 times per day for 5 days.	20 to 40 mg/kg per day divided into 3 daily doses for 5 days.	Severe hepatic or renal impairment, history of gastrointestinal disease, especially colitis.	15.00	Not as effective as tetracycline, especially in nonimmune patients. Used only in combination with a rapidly acting schizonticide such as quinine.
Atovaquone/ proguanil Trade name: Malarone	Treatment of multidrug-resistant *P. falciparum* infections.	4 tablets (1,000 mg atovaquone + 400 mg proguanil) daily for 3 days.	No pediatric formulation currently available, but for patients 11–40 kg in body weight:		35.00	Fixed-dose combination. Reportedly safe in pregnancy and young children. Drug donation program exists. Pediatric formulation in development.

Drug	Indications	Dosage		Value	Comments
Artesunate	Treatment of multidrug-resistant *P. falciparum* infections.	4 mg/kg on day 1 followed by 2 mg/kg daily for total of 7 days.	11-20 kg $^1/_4$ adult dose 21-30 kg $^1/_2$ adult dose 31-40 kg $^3/_4$ adult dose	0.50-1.20	A high number of counterfeit artemisinin products have been found in Southeast Asia.
Artemisinin		20 mg/kg on day 1 followed by 10 mg/kg daily for total of 7 days.	20 mg/kg on day 1 followed by 10 mg/kg daily for total of 7 days.	0.50-2.10	Use of artemisinin derivatives not recommended during first trimester of pregnancy.
Dihydro-artemisinin		4 mg/kg on day 1 followed by 2 mg/ kg daily for total of 7 days.	4 mg/kg on day 1 followed by 2 mg/kg daily for total of 7 days.	?	Rectal preparations of artemisinin and artesunate are available for initial treatment of severe malaria in facilities unable to administer parenteral therapy.

continued

TABLE 3-3 Continued

Drug Name	Use	Dosing (all per os)[a]		Contra-indications	Cost (US$)[b]	Comments
		Adult	Pediatric			
Artemether		4 mg/kg on day 1 followed by 2 mg/kg daily for total of 5 to 7 days.	4 mg/kg on day 1 followed by 2 mg/kg daily for total of 5-7 days.		3.60	
Primaquine	Treatment of *P. vivax* infections (reduce likelihood of relapse). Gametocytocidal agent.	14 mg base per day for 14 days. 45 mg once per week for 8 weeks.	0.3 mg (base)/kg daily for 14 days.	G6PD deficiency, pregnancy.	0.06-0.24	Primaquine has also been investigated for prophylaxis use. See text for additional cautions.

[a] Note: "p.o." or "per os" is latin for "by mouth."
[b] Cost is given for a full adult (60-kg) treatment course. Prices derived from individual reports, personal communications, McFayden (1999), Medical Economics Co. (1999) and WHO (2001b). Prices reflect best prices or best estimates; local prices may differ greatly.

on *P. falciparum* malaria parasites and can no longer be relied on to provide effective treatment or prophylaxis.

Drug resistance is not limited to chloroquine. In some areas of Southeast Asia, the situation is deteriorating to the point where few effective therapies exist. Chloroquine was abandoned as first-line therapy for malaria in Thailand in 1972 in preference to sulfadoxine/pyrimethamine (SP). Drug resistance develops rapidly to dihydrofolate reductase inhibitors (such as pyrimethamine and proguanil) when used alone or in combination with sulfa drugs (such as SP) (Björkman and Phillips-Howard, 1990; Sibley et al., 2001). In 1985, in response to declining SP efficacy, SP was combined with mefloquine (Thaithong et al., 1988). After a few years of widespread use of mefloquine (15 mg/kg), greater than 50 percent of *P. falciparum* infections showed resistance to it in some areas of Thailand (Mockenhaupt, 1995). Cure rates were improved to 70 to 80 percent by increasing the dose of mefloquine to 25 mg/kg, but the efficacy of this higher dose also declined rapidly in some areas (Nosten et al., 2000). In Southeast Asia, parasitological response to quinine has also been deteriorating (Bunnag and Harinasuta, 1987; Wongsrichanalai, et al., 2002). Resistance to newer antimalarials, such as halofantrine, has also been reported, especially in areas with mefloquine resistance (Wongsrichanalai et al., 1992; ter Kuile et al., 1993).

Currently, multidrug-resistant malaria in Thailand is being treated with a combination of an artemisinin derivative and mefloquine; efficacy of this combination has remained high (Nosten et al., 2000). To date, no confirmed cases of resistance to the artemisinin drugs have been reported. However, reports of decreasing sensitivity in vitro in some areas, as well as a number of case reports of potential (but unconfirmed) treatment failures, raise concern that this class of antimalarial drug is not "immune" to the development of resistance (Wongsrichanalai et al., 1999; Sahr et al., 2001).

In many areas where population displacement occurs, national treatment policies of the host and source countries may not necessarily reflect the drug resistance patterns of a given region or population. In many cases this is due to a lack of current efficacy data, a lack of funds for implementation of a new policy, and a variety of other concerns (Bloland and Ettling, 1999). For example, CQ is still the recommended first-line treatment for *P. falciparum* in much of Africa, despite the high prevalence of CRPF. Choice of the most appropriate antimalarial drug should be based, whenever possible, on actual evaluation of the efficacy of possible therapeutic options using standard methods (see Appendix B).

Drug resistance is not an all-or-nothing phenomenon. In any given area, a wide range of parasitological responses can be found, from complete sensitivity to high-level resistance (see Table 3-4). In general, malaria parasites in western sub-Saharan Africa are less resistant to drugs like CQ and SP than malaria parasites in eastern or southern Africa. In Southeast Asia the distribution of drug resistance is highly variable and focal. While some very well-publicized areas (such as the refugee camps along the Thai-Burmese border) are faced with highly resistant malaria, requiring complicated combination therapy approaches, nearby areas reportedly have had a much longer period of success with MQ alone (K. Thimasarn, Malaria Control Programme, Thai Ministry of Public Health, 1998, personal communication; Singhasivanon, 1999; Wongsrichanalai et al., 2000).

The policy response to increasing evidence of antimalarial drug resistance has been variable as well. In parts of East Africa, parasitological resistance to CQ is very high, with 80 to 90 percent of *P. falciparum* infections being moderately to highly resistant (Bloland et al., 1993). In response to these high rates of resistance, Malawi switched from CQ to SP for first-line therapy for *P. falciparum* in 1993. A number of countries in eastern and southern Africa (including Tanzania, Kenya, Democratic Republic of Congo, Rwanda, Uganda, Ethiopia) have made similar policy changes to SP alone or in combination (with either CQ or amodiaquine) on a national or provincial/district level. After a long period of disinclination to change treatment policies, many more countries in sub-Saharan Africa are now reevaluating their national treatment guidelines and considering policy changes to locally effective regimens. Although the drugs being used differ, similar efforts are under way in the Amazon region and Southeast Asia.

VECTOR CONTROL

Attempts to interfere with the entomological link in malaria transmission are an essential and integral part of many malaria control programs. However, a vector control measure that is appropriate in one setting may be totally inappropriate elsewhere (see earlier section on Malaria Vectors and Vector Behavior). It is therefore strongly advised that the assistance of an experienced medical entomologist who is familiar with existing malaria vector data for the area in question be obtained. Decisions based on expert advice and firsthand data are the most certain route to cost-effective vector control.

The importance of understanding vector biology and behavior prior to initiating control measures is evident when one considers the key questions that must be answered to determine which type of control measure is best for a given situation. Identification of the mosquito species responsible for most malaria transmission involves surveillance, collection, and species identification from various parts of the affected area. There can also be a number of anophelines in a given area. However, not all anopheline mosquitoes transmit malaria and not all anophelines that do transmit malaria are efficient vectors. Therefore, the most commonly collected adult anopheline species captured in a given area will sometimes, but not always, be responsible for most malaria transmission. Control activities aimed at one important vector species may not be effective against another vector species. For example, insecticide-treated nets may be useful for reducing exposure to mosquitoes biting inside houses but may have no effect on mosquitoes biting primarily outside.

Information about the breeding places of vectors is required. Mosquitoes have diverse breeding habits, some of which may be targeted for control purposes. Mosquitoes generally do not range farther than 2 to 3 km from their breeding sites, unless carried by winds or some other vehicle. When one site or a few produce most of the vectors responsible for transmission, larval control may be appropriate and effective. In situations where breeding sites are small, dispersed, or not easily identified, however, larval control would be inappropriate. As mentioned previously, some malaria vectors (such as *An. gambiae* in Africa) can breed in pools as small and temporary as an animal's hoofprint. Identifying breeding areas also requires considerable skill. When done correctly, larval control has been very effective in certain circumstances, such as special projects, urban areas, and land-based business ventures.

Differences in the behavior patterns of adult mosquitoes have a marked effect on their capacity to transmit malaria as well as the choice of control methods used. Preferred time of biting, for example, can vary from daytime to late evening. The efficacy of many control measures varies, depending on the mosquito activity cycle. Insecticide-treated bed nets or other control measures that are used indoors, such as space spraying with insecticides, would obviously have little effect on malaria transmission occurring at times when people are not indoors. For example, malaria transmission in much of Southeast Asia is associated with exposure to mosquitoes during activities conducted in the forest.

TABLE 3-4 Distribution of Drug-Resistant *P. falciparum* Malaria.

Region	Resistance Reported[1]			
	CQ	SP	MQ	Others
Central America (Mexico, Belize, Guatemala, Honduras, El Salvador, Nicaragua, Costa Rica, Northwestern Panama)	N	N	N	
Carribean (Haiti and Dominican Republic only)	N	N	N	
South America (Southeastern Panama, Columbia, Venezuela, Ecuador, Peru, Brazil, Bolivia)	F	F	R	QN
West Africa	F	R	R	
East Africa	F	R	R	
Southern Africa	F	F/R	N	
Indian subcontinent	F	R	N	
Southeast Asia and Oceania	F	F	F	HAL, QN
East Asia (China)	F	F	F	

NOTES: [1]Reports of resistance to a given agent occurring in an area do not necessarily mean that occurrence is frequent enough to pose a significant public health risk. "F" indicates agents to which frequent resistance occurs in a given area (although actual risk may be highly focal—e.g., Southeast Asia, where MQ resistance, while very frequent in

Comments

Northwest of Panama Canal only.

Resistance to MQ and QN, although reported, is considered to occur infrequently.

Incidence of resistance to CQ is variable but very common in most areas.

Incidence of resistance to SP is highly variable, with some reports of high levels occurring focally but generally low to moderate.

Resistance to SP is considered to be generally low, except for KwaZulu Natal Province, South Africa; MQ resistance is probably very rare (reported from Malawi).

Border areas of Thailand, Cambodia, and Myanmar at highest risk for multidrug-resistant infections; in other areas, incidence of resistance to SP and MQ is highly variable or even absent.

Greatest problem with resistance in southern China where bulk of falciparum transmission occurs.

some limited areas, is infrequent or absent in most others). "R" indicates that, while resistance to agent has been reported and can be focally common, it is not believed to occur frequently enough to warrant complete avoidance of that particular drug. "N" indicates that resistance has not been reported to date or occurs at a rate low enough to not present a substantial public health threat.

Technical Overview of the Epidemiology of Malaria: Key Points

- Technical knowledge about malaria will assist in making a determination as to whether malaria poses a significant threat during a complex emergency.

- Malaria occurs primarily in tropical and some subtropical regions of Africa, Central and South America, Asia, and Oceania.

- There is tremendous geographic variation in intensity of transmission and risk of infection.

- Human malaria is caused by one or more parasites: *Plasmodium falciparum*, *P. vivax*, *P. ovale*, or *P. malariae*. *P. falciparum* is most closely associated with fatal malaria.

- Malaria is most commonly transmitted by the bite of an infected female *Anopheles* mosquito. Other major ways malaria is transmitted are through blood transfusions and transplacentally.

- Not all *Anopheles* mosquitoes are malaria vectors, and not all vector species transmit malaria equally well.

- Vector behavior varies considerably by species throughout the world in regard to malaria.

- Understanding the implications of vector behavior helps in identifying appropriate vector control strategies for a specific area.

- Malaria has nonspecific symptoms and is difficult to distinguish clinically from other febrile illnesses.

- Partial immunity to malaria is acquired after repeated exposure and infection.

- In order to estimate the potential impact of malaria in a given population it is important to understand the relationship between transmission intensity, levels of acquired immunity within a population, and manifestations of malaria illness.

- Certain groups are considered to be highly vulnerable populations, especially pregnant women and very young children.

- Malaria during pregnancy can be the cause of substantial maternal and fetal/infant morbidity and mortality.

- The important clinical consequences of malaria during pregnancy differ given the underlying level of acquired immunity.

- Among nonimmune pregnant women, malaria can cause severe illness, fetal loss, or maternal death.

- Among semiimmune pregnant women, malaria can cause substantial maternal anemia and low birth weight.

- Antimalarial drug resistance is rapidly increasing, both in terms of the number of drugs involved and the areas of the world in which it is occurring.

- Local malaria treatment guidelines and policies are frequently out of date with regard to the current status of antimalarial drug resistance.

- Vector control strategies need to reflect an understanding of both vector biology and behavior.

- Expert entomological advice is often needed to identify the most appropriate antivector interventions.

4

Essential Components/Design of an Optimal Malaria Control Program

A basic malaria control program combines five components: a public health surveillance system, curative services, preventive interventions, a program for community involvement, and a capacity to perform special studies (operational research) as needed. Briefly, a *public health surveillance system* is required to monitor temporal changes in disease incidence, to warn of epidemics, and to evaluate the impact of control efforts. This is obviously important for more than just malaria, and a well-designed and integrated surveillance system provides an essential tool for monitoring a rapidly changeable health situation. *Curative services* include the provision of prompt diagnosis of malaria and an assessment of its severity, diagnosis of malaria-associated anemia and other potential consequences of the disease, and prompt and effective treatment of both malaria and anemia. *Preventive interventions* are essential for limiting malaria-associated morbidity and mortality that would not be achievable through curative services alone. Prevention would include some combination of preventive use of antimalarial drugs, encouraging use of personal protection measures, introducing insecticide-treated bed nets, and vector control. The success or failure of any public health program is determined in large part by the public's acceptance and proper use of the services offered. Therefore, a program to establish a high degree of *community involvement* is an important, albeit often underappreciated, component of a malaria control program. Finally, agencies should develop a capacity to conduct simple *operational research* to answer specific questions, to evaluate the impact of interventions, to improve the implementation of interventions, and to test novel approaches to implementing specific interventions.

5

Public Health Surveillance System

A fundamental tool that must be included in any approach to the problem of controlling communicable diseases following mass population movements for any cause is a public health surveillance system. A well-designed surveillance system allows for rapid identification of increases in cases of communicable diseases in an affected area, signaling the need for a specific response. Basic demographic data should be collected, in addition to simple case counts using standardized case definitions. These include age, sex, pregnancy status, location of residence in the settlement area, and so forth. These data can be used to identify high-risk subgroups in the general population or areas in a settlement that might require specific attention (e.g., previously unrecognized vector breeding sites).

Another aspect of surveillance that is often overlooked is ongoing monitoring of first-line antimalarial drug efficacy among the affected population. Drug efficacy can change dramatically over relatively short periods of time, especially in areas where antimalarial drugs are easily obtainable in the community. Periodic monitoring (at least once every two years and in some situations as often as once a year) of the drugs used for first-line treatment of malaria should be a priority. Monitoring in-hospital case fatality rates can aid in the early recognition of declining efficacy of second- or third-line antimalarial drugs as well as identify other operational problems with the management of malaria patients.

PRACTICAL CONSIDERATIONS FOR SURVEILLANCE SYSTEMS

The success of a surveillance system rests on the availability of a functional communication and logistical infrastructure that allows for timely information transfer among all users of the system. For surveillance systems to be effective, the flow of information must occur in two directions—the data must be fed into the surveillance system and a practical interpretation of the data must be returned to the health care workers. Health care workers need to receive timely feedback on the statistics they are collecting in order to make policy or programmatic decisions, particularly if there is suspicion of a pending epidemic. Additionally, if information mostly flows into the system and little or no information is returned, enthusiasm for collecting and reporting quality data will wane, jeopardizing the validity and usefulness of the system. The Centers for Disease Control and Prevention (2001) published a useful guide to evaluating surveillance systems.

Many health care workers in refugee camps have minimal training and do not understand the importance of malaria surveillance; therefore, it is wise to spend time training workers not only in how to systematically collect data but also about the potential impact these data can make in case management. For example, in the Thai/Myanmar border camps, a medic who received such training was able to rapidly detect an epidemic. Because the supervising nongovernmental organization physician was only able to visit the camp intermittently, not having well-trained and motivated camp staff might have led to a much larger outbreak (MacArthur et al., 2001).

STANDARDIZED CASE DEFINITIONS[1]

A primary problem facing malaria surveillance is the choice of a single case definition and obtaining agreement on standardized reporting of data, especially in situations where multiple NGOs are providing health care services. Without standardized case definitions and reporting systems, the ability to produce reliable interpretation of surveillance data to determine disease trends in an affected population is questionable.

Wherever possible, malaria cases should be confirmed using an accepted laboratory test (such as examination of blood slides). Commercially made rapid diagnostic tests for malaria are available and could be

---

[1]See also Diagnosis of Malaria in Chapter 6.

used but currently are cost prohibitive in many settings. Besides improving the specificity of reporting, the use of microscopy will identify patients with nonmalarial febrile disease requiring further investigation, identify patients with nonfalciparum malaria, identify patients with hyper-parasitemia, and reduce the amount of inappropriate antimalarial drug use.

In circumstances where routine microscopic diagnosis is not possible, such as situations where health care facilities are unable to perform microscopy or lack the capacity to keep up with the patient load (a frequent situation in the acute phase of an emergency), a simple clinical case definition can be used. A commonly used definition is "fever or history of fever in the absence of an obvious cause." The use of clinical case definitions, however, will overestimate the incidence of malaria. Surveillance systems that rely on clinical case definitions should be complemented with periodic blood slide surveys of patients meeting this definition to aid in the interpretation of surveillance data.

Public Health Surveillance System: Key Points

- Effective surveillance is essential for monitoring disease trends and providing early warnings of potential epidemics or increasing drug resistance.

- Ongoing monitoring of first-line antimalarial drug efficacy should be a routine form of surveillance for the affected population (see special studies).

- A functional communication system and logistical infrastructure is necessary for timely information transfer between participating facilities or organizations.

- To be useful as feedback for clinical management decisions, surveillance information should be summarized and returned to clinical services in an efficient manner.

RECOMMENDATIONS

Our main recommendations for policy makers and field staff are:

- Ensure that a functional surveillance system for communicable diseases is operational as early in an emergency situation as possible.
- Provide necessary training in the use of surveillance information for all health care and administrative workers involved with surveillance.
- Require standardization in case definitions and forms used by all agencies.
- Establish a system for ongoing drug efficacy monitoring of first-line antimalarial therapy.
- Provide timely feedback to health care agencies summarizing the implications of the surveillance data.

6

Curative Services:
Malaria Therapy and Case Management

Effective case management is the minimum requirement for any malaria control program. Because falciparum malaria can become life threatening within just 48 hours, first-line therapy needs to be offered at the most peripheral facilities. A system of referral needs to be established so that patients requiring more aggressive therapy for severe disease can get to a central facility where appropriate care can be given, such as parenteral antimalarials and supportive care. Health care providers in central locations need to be trained and able to deliver both specific and supportive care to unconscious malaria patients.

As mentioned previously, the choice of drugs used for uncomplicated severe malaria at different levels of the health care system must be based on relevant data regarding drug resistance patterns and expected efficacy. Occasionally, sufficient information can be obtained from the host country or existing literature; however, specific drug efficacy studies conducted with standard methods in the population being served are the best way to determine the most appropriate drugs to use. Simple methods for assessing the efficacy of first-line antimalarial drugs are presented in Appendix B. Currently, standardized in vivo efficacy studies are rarely conducted during the acute phase of an emergency; however, these data are necessary in order to make decisions regarding effective malaria treatment. Often nongovernmental organizations (NGOs) are overburdened by the demands of providing essential services or lack staff members with experience in conducting such studies. The Roll Back Malaria Technical Resource Network for Malaria Control in Complex Emergencies is an example of a resource for technical assistance in this area (see Appendix D for more information on resources).

DIAGNOSIS OF MALARIA

A number of options exist or are in development for diagnosing malaria (see Table 6-1). The most common methods of diagnosis are either those based on clinical signs and symptoms alone or those based on microscopy. Newer technologies, especially rapid diagnostic tests, are becoming more widely used. Cost and prevailing conditions (availability of electricity, equipment, supplies, adequate training, and supervision) typically determine the method used. In Africa, for instance, clinical diagnosis of malaria is most commonly used, both in complex emergency situations and stable populations. Rapid diagnostic tests have rarely been used operationally in complex emergencies. When they have been used, it is usually in conjunction with rapid surveys rather than routine diagnosis (Kassankogno et al., 2000).

METHODS OF DIAGNOSIS

Clinical (Presumptive) Diagnosis

Although reliable diagnosis cannot be made on the basis of signs and symptoms alone because of the nonspecific nature of clinical malaria, clinical diagnosis of malaria is common in many malarious areas. In much of the malaria-endemic world, resources and trained health care personnel are so scarce that presumptive clinical diagnosis is the only realistic option and is a common approach in the context of complex emergencies, especially in sub-Saharan Africa. Clinical diagnosis offers the advantages of ease, speed, and low cost. In areas where malaria is prevalent, clinical diagnosis usually results in all patients with fever and no other apparent cause being treated for malaria. This approach can identify most patients who truly need antimalarial treatment but is also likely to misclassify many who do not (Olivar et al., 1991). Overdiagnosis can be considerable and contributes to misuse of antimalarial drugs, places individuals at unnecessary risk of side effects, and can contribute to the development of drug resistance. Considerable overlap exists between the signs and symptoms of malaria and other common diseases, especially acute lower respiratory tract infections and acute viral syndromes, and can greatly increase the frequency of misdiagnosis and mistreatment (Redd et al., 1992; Rey et al., 1996).

Attempts to improve the specificity of clinical diagnosis for malaria by including signs and symptoms other than fever or history of fever have met with only minimal success (Smith et al., 1994). The Integrated Management of Childhood Illnesses (IMCI) is a strategy developed to improve diagnosis and treatment of the most common childhood illnesses in areas that must rely on relatively unskilled health care workers without access to laboratories or special equipment. With this strategy, every febrile child living in a "high-risk" area for malaria is considered to have, and is treated for, malaria (although many children will likely be treated for other illnesses as well). "High risk" is defined in the IMCI Adaptation Guides as being any situation where as little as 5 percent of febrile children between the ages of 2 and 59 months are parasitemic (World Health Organization, 1997a), a definition that will likely lead to significant overdiagnosis of malaria in areas with low-to-moderate malaria transmission. Although this strategy may improve diagnosis of childhood illnesses, it requires substantial investment in training and supervision. Its usefulness in a complex emergency will likely be contingent on the relief agency's commitment to sustain this level of effort.

Laboratory-Based Diagnosis

Wherever possible, laboratory-based diagnosis should be used. It offers the advantage of identifying not only patients truly in need of malaria treatment but also patients who do not and who should therefore be reassessed for another cause of their fever. By reducing unnecessary malaria treatment, overall drug pressure on the parasite, an important contributing factor in the development of drug resistance, can also be reduced.

Although laboratory-based diagnosis is typically more expensive and labor intensive than clinical diagnosis, it has been shown to be cost effective in some settings and can potentially lower actual malaria treatment costs by reducing the amounts of antimalarial drugs that are used. This is especially true in settings where inexpensive antimalarials, such as chloroquine and sulfadoxine/pyrimethamine, can no longer be used because of high levels of drug resistance.

Species diagnosis is another important advantage to laboratory-based diagnosis. In most areas of the world, nonfalciparum malaria can be reliably

TABLE 6-1 Comparative Descriptions of Available Malaria
Diagnostic Methods

Method	Sensitivity/Specificity[a]	Advantages
Clinical, especially based on formal algorithm such as Integrated Management of Childhood Illnesses (IMCI) or similar algorithm	Variable depending on level of clinical competency, training, and malaria risk (endemicity): with IMCI: low risk: sens: 87% spec: 8% high risk: sens: 100% spec: 0%	Speed and ease of use. No electricity or special equipment needed beyond normal clinical equipment (thermometer, stethoscope, otoscope, timer).
Light microscopy	Optimal conditions: sens: >90% spec: 100% Typical field conditions: sens: 25-100% spec: 56-100%	Species-specific diagnosis. Quantification of parasitemia aids treatment follow-up.
Flourescent microscopy: • Acridine orange (AO) stained thick blood smears	AO: sens: 42-93% spec: 52-93%	Results attainable more quickly than normal microscopy.
• Quantitative Buffy Coat (QBC; Becton-Dickinson)	QBC: sens: 89% spec: >95%	
Rapid diagnostic stick test based on PfHRP-II (various tests and manufacturers)	sens: 84-97% spec: 81-100% Lower values probably due to low parasite densities.	Speed and ease of use; minimal training requirements to achieve reliable results. No electricity or special equipment needed. Could be used at health post/community outreach. Card format easier to use for individual tests; dipstick test easier to use for batched testing.

Disadvantages	Cost[b]	References
Can result in high degree of misdiagnosis and overtreatment for malaria. Requires close supervision and retraining to maximize reliability. Algorithm increases time spent with each patient if done correctly, requiring substantial staffing to implement in areas with high patient load.	Variable depending on situation.	Olivar (1991) Sowunmi and Akindele (1993) Weber et al. (1996) Perkins et al. (1997) Bojang et al. (2000)
Requires relatively high degree of training and supervision for reliable results. Sensitivity and specificity dependent on training and supervision. Special equipment and supplies needed. Electricity desirable. Time consuming.	0.03-0.08[c]	Craig and Sharp (1997) Barat et al. (1999)
Special equipment and supplies needed. Sensitivity of AO poor with low parasite densities. Electricity required. Unreliable species diagnosis; nonspecific staining of debris and nonparasitic cells. QBC will not quantify parsitemia. AO is a hazardous material.	0.03 (AO)- 1.70 (QBC)	Makler et al. (1998) Craig and Sharp (1997)
Will not diagnose nonfalciparum malaria, although subsequent-generation tests will be able to do this. Will not quantify parsitemia (+/- only). Can remain positive after clearance of parasites.	0.80-1.00	World Health Organization (1996c) Craig and Sharp (1997)

continued

TABLE 6-1 Continued

Method	Sensitivity/Specificity[a]	Advantages
Rapid diagnostic test based on pLDH: (OptiMal, Flow, Inc.)	sens: 81-100% spec: 100%	Differentiates *P. falciparum* from nonfalciparum infections. Speed and ease of use; minimal training requirements to achieve reliable result. Reportedly does not remain positive after clearance of parasites. No electricity or special equipment needed. Could be used in community outreach programs.

[a] Sensitivity (sens) or the proportion of true positives that are identified as positive by test; specificity (spec) or the proportion of true negatives identified as negative by the test.
[b] Approximate or projected cost given in U.S. dollars per test performed; reflects only the cost of expendable materials unless otherwise noted.

treated with chloroquine alone or chloroquine and primaquine, reducing overall malaria treatment costs while ensuring appropriate treatment of falciparum malaria.

Microscopy

Simple light microscopic examination of (preferably) Giemsa-stained blood films is the most widely practiced and useful method for definitive malaria diagnosis. Advantages include differentiation between species, quantification of parasite density, and the ability to distinguish clinically important asexual parasite stages from gametocytes, which may persist without causing symptoms. These advantages can also be critical for proper case management. For example, the ability to quantify parasite density offers a method to evaluate parasitological response to treatment, which is needed for early identification of treatment failure. The disadvantages are

Disadvantages	Cost[b]	References
Cannot differentiate between nonfalciparum species. Will not quantify parsitemia (+/- only). Sensitivity declines with very low parasitemias (i.e., < 50 parasites/mm^3).	1.00	Piper et al. (1999) Makler et al. (1998)

[c]Cost includes salaries of microscopists and expendable supplies; does not include cost of training, supervision, or equipment.
SOURCES: Table modified from Stennies (1999) and Centers for Disease Control and Prevention unpublished document.

that slide collection, staining, and reading can be time consuming, and microscopists need to be trained and supervised to ensure consistent reliability. While the availability of microscopic diagnosis has been shown to reduce drug use in some trial settings (Jonkman et al., 1995), in practice the results are often unreliable or disregarded by clinicians (Barat et al., 1999). Any program aimed at improving the availability of reliable microscopy should also retrain clinicians in the use and interpretation of microscopic diagnosis.

A second method is a modification of light microscopy called the quantitative buffy coat method (QBC, by Becton-Dickenson). Originally developed to screen large numbers of specimens for complete blood cell counts, this method has been adapted for malaria diagnosis (Levine et al., 1989). The technique uses microhematocrit tubes precoated with flourescent acridine orange stain to highlight malaria parasites. With centrifugation, parasites are concentrated at a predictable location. Advantages to QBC are that less training is required to operate the system than for reading Giemsa-stained blood films, and the test is typically quicker to perform than normal light microscopy. Field trials have shown that the QBC system may be marginally more sensitive than conventional microscopy under ideal conditions (Rickman et al., 1989; Tharavanij, 1990). Disadvantages are that electricity is always required, special equipment and supplies are needed, the per-test cost is higher than simple light microscopy, and species-specific diagnosis is not reliable. This methodology is currently used infrequently and supplies are increasingly difficult to locate.

Rapid Diagnostic Tests

A third diagnostic approach involves the rapid detection of parasite antigens using rapid immunochromatographic techniques (also known as "dipstick" tests). Multiple experimental tests have been developed targeting a variety of parasite antigens (Mackey et al., 1982; Fortier et al., 1987; Khusmith et al., 1987). A number of commercially available kits are based on the detection of the histidine-rich protein 2 (HRP-II) of *P. falciparum*. Compared with light microscopy and QBC, this test yields rapid and highly sensitive diagnosis of *P. falciparum* infection (World Health Organization, 1996b; Craig and Sharp, 1997). Advantages to this technology are that no special equipment is required, only minimal training is necessary and no electricity is needed. The principal disadvantages are the currently high per-test cost and an inability to quantify the density of infection. Furthermore, for tests based on HRP-II, detectable antigen can persist for days after adequate treatment and cure; therefore, the test cannot adequately distinguish a resolving infection from treatment failure due to drug resistance, especially early after treatment (World Health Organization, 1996b). Additionally, a test based on detection of a specific parasite enzyme (lactate dehydrogenase or pLDH) has been developed (OptiMAL, by Flow, Inc., Portland, Oregon). It reportedly detects only viable parasites, which, if true, eliminates prolonged periods of false positivity posttreatment (Makler et al., 1998; Piper et al., 1999; Palmer et al., 1999). Newer-generation antigen detection tests are able to distinguish between falciparum and nonfalciparum infections, greatly expanding their usefulness in areas where nonfalciparum malaria is transmitted frequently. Finally, there is growing concern about the stability, shelf life, and reliability of these tests under field conditions. Exposure to heat and humidity have been raised as possible factors that could compromise test function (L. Causer, Centers for Disease

Control and Prevention, personal communication, 2002). For a more complete review of rapid diagnostic tests for malaria, see Moody (2002).

Molecular Tests

Detection of parasite genetic material or resistance-conferring mutations through polymerase chain reaction techniques is becoming a more frequently used tool in the diagnosis of malaria, as well as the diagnosis and surveillance of drug resistance in malaria (Plowe et al., 1995). At present, however, this method of diagnosis is well beyond the capacity of most NGOs or relief agencies. Since sample collection is exceedingly easy (a dried blood spot on filter paper), collaboration with an outside agency or ministry of health that does have this capacity would allow its use for monitoring patterns of resistance to chloroquine or sulfadoxine/pyrimethamine in an emergency setting, particularly in areas where in vivo studies would be difficult to conduct. This approach is being used to supplement in vivo drug efficacy testing in the Democratic Republic of Congo (P. Bloland, Centers for Disease Control and Prevention, unpublished data, 2001). This methodology has limitations, however. Because samples must be analyzed in specialized laboratories, it may take months to obtain results. Mutations related to resistance have been identified only for chloroquine, sulfadoxine/pyrimethamine, and atovaquone. Finally, although the relationship between the presence of resistance-conferring mutations and clinical or parasitological response to treatment has been investigated (Djimdé et al., 2001), it probably differs from location to location depending on underlying levels of immunity in the population and the specific drug being tested.

The method to be used to diagnose malaria is an important issue for consideration when setting up malaria control programs. Not all situations will allow for definitive diagnosis, such as facilities seeing very high volumes of patients, community outreach programs, or during epidemics. At a minimum, some form of laboratory-based diagnosis (most likely microscopy) should be available in all situations as an aid in the diagnosis and management of severe malaria. However, the decision to use laboratory tests (as well as the decision of which diagnostic tests to use) for routine diagnosis of all suspected malaria cases needs to be based on:

- patient load;
- time required to do the test;
- cost of the test;

- cost savings that might be expected from avoiding unnecessary malaria treatment;
- level of training and supervision of laboratory and clinical staff and number of trained staff members available; and
- availability of electricity, appropriate equipment, and supplies.

In typical relief efforts in Africa, patient load alone makes the use of laboratory-based diagnosis difficult. In western Tanzania, for instance, although microscopy was available, it was used only for diagnosis of malaria among inpatients, staff, or particularly confusing cases (e.g., to help decide between malaria and an acute lower respiratory tract infection; H. Williams and P. Bloland, Centers for Disease Control and Prevention, unpublished data, 1998). Because the microscopes relied on sunlight, no microscopy was available on particularly cloudy days or during evening hours. The majority of patients were diagnosed using clinical impressions alone. While rapid diagnostic tests could have been used in this setting, the current cost of these tests would have been prohibitive for the budgets of most NGOs.

TREATMENT OF MALARIA

Prompt provision of effective therapy that is capable of preventing the progression of illness from mild to severe has been estimated to provide as much as a 50-fold reduction in the risk of mortality. In contrast, effective treatment of malaria once it has progressed to severe illness has only a five-fold reduction in the probability of dying (White, 1999). Mortality among patients being treated for severe or cerebral malaria in a hospital is 10 to 40 percent, even when the best treatment is given (Greenberg et al., 1989; Molyneux et al., 1989). Progression of death can be rapid; the mean time between onset of illness and death among Gambian children was 2.8 days (Greenwood et al., 1987).

Treatment of Uncomplicated *P. falciparum* Malaria

The choice of an optimal treatment regimen for uncomplicated malaria depends on local drug resistance patterns, acceptability (in terms of safety, side effects, ability to use during pregnancy, ability to treat young children), and cost. Other considerations in choosing a treatment regimen for a given situation include the need to train or retrain staff, ease of administration, probable adherence to recommended dosing regimen, and an assured supply of drugs.

Combinations of artemisinin derivatives (such as 3 days of artesunate and another common antimalarial drug, such as mefloquine, sulfadoxine/ pyrimethamine, or amodiaquine) are currently being evaluated as options for treating uncomplicated *P. falciparum* malaria. Artemisinin (ART) derivatives produce rapid killing of parasites, greatly reducing the parasite load. Because ART derivatives must be used for 7 days when used alone, combination with a second drug allows fewer days of treatment (3 days) while maintaining high efficacy, thus improving compliance. In specific areas of low transmission in Southeast Asia, ART combination therapy appears to have slowed the development of drug resistance and possibly decreased malaria transmission (Price et al., 1997; Nosten et al., 2000).

Although the combination of ART and mefloquine has been used extensively and successfully in refugee camps in Thailand (as well as in stable populations in parts of Southeast Asia), there has been very limited experience with the programmatic use (for either displaced or stable populations) of this or other ART combinations in Africa or the Americas, although preliminary studies and evaluations are being conducted (Doherty et al., 1999; von Seidlein et al., 2000; Bloland et al., 2000; Kachur et al., 2001).

Two often-cited reasons to use an ART combination treatment strategy—inhibition of development of resistance and reduction in malaria transmission rates—are unproven in areas of moderate-to-intense malaria transmission, such as is found in most of tropical Africa (Price et al., 1996; White et al., 1999; Bloland et al., 2000). Nonetheless, ART in combination with a second drug appropriate to the region would probably offer optimum efficacy. If these additional properties of artemisinin-containing combination therapy (ACT) are proven, a strong argument could be made to preferentially use such combinations to protect antimalarial drugs and to reduce malaria transmission, an especially desirable effect during an epidemic. Presently, however, the decision to utilize ACT, especially in areas of moderate-to-high transmission, should be based on comparison between ACT and other available malaria drugs in terms of efficacy, availability, cost, effectiveness, and other operational factors and not on unproven characteristics. Other available therapeutic options are presented in Appendix A and Table 3-3. Not all of the options presented would be appropriate, however, for any given setting or situation. Additionally, some drug choices that would appear optimal in the context of a complex emergency may conflict with the national malaria treatment policy of the host country. Many national malaria treatment policies lag behind current status of drug resistance, especially in Africa. Nonetheless, ministries of health may require evidence that the prevailing national treatment policy is inadequate to treat refugee populations before allowing a deviation from national policy. For example, prior to 1999 in refugee camps in western Tanzania, the first-line treatment for uncomplicated malaria was chloroquine in accordance with the national treatment guidelines. Faced with increasing reports of chloroquine failures, standardized in vivo studies were conducted in the camps and surrounding communities. Based on these data, a decision was made to allow sulfadoxine/pyrimethamine to be used for first-line therapy in the camps, even though chloroquine continued to be recommended for the national population (H. Williams, Centers for Disease Control and Prevention, unpublished data, 1999).

As mentioned, drug resistance patterns can be highly variable within relatively small geographic areas, and predictions of likely therapeutic efficacy based on the geographic location of the area in which a displaced population settles may prove to be inaccurate. Although some generalizations can be made (see Table 3-4), more accurate information should be obtained through operational research or from reliable local or international sources.

Treatment of Nonfalciparum Malaria

Chloroquine remains a highly effective treatment for nonfalciparum infections in most areas of the world. In areas where nonfalciparum malaria infections are relatively common, distinguishing nonfalciparum infections from falciparum infections could result in cost savings, especially if treatment of falciparum infections is expensive. Primaquine reduces the probability of relapse due to *P. vivax* and *P. ovale;* in situations where rapid reinfection with *P. vivax* or *P. ovale* or poor compliance with a 14-day regimen is likely, however, use of primaquine as a routine antirelapse treatment is often not a priority. Nonetheless, data from areas of relatively low transmission suggest that routine use of 14 days of primaquine (but not less) could potentially prevent a substantial amount of febrile illness and anemia associated with preventable relapses of *P. vivax* (Luxemberger et al., 1999; Rowland and Durrani, 1999).

Chloroquine-resistant *P. vivax* has been reported to occur at low levels in some regions. In some locations it can occur frequently enough to raise questions about the wisdom of continued use of the drug, such as Irian Jaya, Indonesia, and Papua New Guinea (Murphy et al., 1993). In areas where chloroquine-resistant vivax is common, such infections should be treated as for chloroquine-resistant falciparum. However, some drugs that can be used for *P. falciparum* are not optimally effective for *P. vivax*, especially sulfadoxine/pyrimethamine (Pukrittayakamee et al., 2000a).

Some geographic areas have *P. vivax* parasites with a reduced sensitivity to primaquine. This is particularly true of vivax infections from Southeast Asia and Oceania (Collins and Jeffery, 1996). These infections can sometimes be successfully treated using 30 mg daily for 14 days, rather than the standard 15-mg daily regimen adult dose. A new drug related to primaquine (tafenoquine; see Table 3-3) is being developed that offers increased efficacy and may replace primaquine in the treatment of *P. vivax* (Walsh et al., 1999).

Primaquine can cause severe or fatal hemolysis in patients with G6PD deficiencies. Populations with certain ethnic backgrounds are at increased risk of severe G6PD deficiency and therefore increased risk of hemolysis. Severe deficiency (<10 percent residual enzyme activity) is seen in some people of Mediterranean and Asian decent; moderate deficiency (10 to 60 percent residual activity) is common among populations of African descent. Ideally, all patients needing primaquine treatment should be tested for G6PD deficiency before treatment begins, but in a complex emergency this rarely occurs. Patients with severe deficiency (and any pregnant women) should not receive primaquine; most patients with moderate deficiency (African A variant) can be treated with a larger dose of primaquine

Caution on Primaquine Use

CAUTION: Primaquine can cause severe or potentially fatal hemolysis in patients with a deficiency in the enzyme glucose-6-phosphate dehydrogenase (G6PD). Risk and severity of G6PD deficiency vary with ethnicity. Primaquine should not be used during pregnancy.

less often (45 mg primaquine base orally once a week for 8 weeks for adults) without producing life-threatening hemolysis.

Treatment of Severe Falciparum Malaria

Treatment of severe *P. falciparum* malaria should be with immediate administration of parental quinine or quinidine, beginning with a loading dose and followed by 8 to 12 hourly maintenance doses (World Health Organization, 2000a, 2000b). This regimen should be continued until the patient can take oral medications. Quality nursing care and close clinical monitoring are essential, especially for comatose patients.

Quinine remains the standard treatment for severe malaria illness because of its ready availability, efficacy, and rapid action. While artemisinins have been used for the treatment of severe malaria, there is no clear indication that they are superior to quinine in terms of patient survival (World Health Organization, 2000a). However, in areas where quinine resistance is known to occur, artemisinins offer obvious advantages.

Quinine use is often restricted to facilities that have the capacity to carefully monitor patients for potential cardiac side effects from the quinine therapy and to properly administer and monitor intravenous fluids and medicines. Another consideration, therefore, that might favor the use of artemisinins in the context of complex emergencies is a lack of capacity of facilities to administer parenteral quinine safely and effectively. Patients with severe falciparum malaria being managed at facilities with minimal capacity could potentially be treated with an artemisinin suppository before being transferred to a better-equipped and better-staffed facility for complete management (Krishna et al., 2001). Alternatively, if a facility has the capacity to provide injections but not intravenous therapy, patients could be treated with either artemether or artesunate intramuscularly. Dosing with artemisinin or artesunate intramuscularly can be done on a once-daily basis, greatly increasing the ease of treatment. (See Appendix C for recommendations for possible alternative regimens.) Of note, some large studies of artemisinin use for treating patients with severe falciparum malaria have noted delayed resolution of coma; the reasons and implications of this delayed recovery are unknown (World Health Organization, 2000a).

Nursing Care for Severe Malaria

Severely ill malaria patients, especially those who are comatose, require

Recommended Regimen for Treatment of Severe Malaria

Loading dose: Quinine dihydrochloride 20 mg (salt)/kg of body weight infused over 4 hours in 5 percent dextrose saline (5 to 10 mg/kg body weight depending on the patient's overall fluid balance).

Maintenance doses: Quinine dihydrochloride 10 mg (salt)/kg of body weight infused over 4 hours in 5 percent dextrose saline (5 to 10 mg/kg body weight depending on the patient's overall fluid balance) starting 8 to 12 hours after the start of the loading dose. Repeat this maintenance dose every 8 to 12 hours (from start of previous dose) until patient can take oral medications. Among patients requiring intravenous therapy for longer than 48 hours, doses of quinine should be reduced by one-third to one-half starting on the third day of treatment.

Subsequent oral dosing: As soon as the patient is able to take oral medications, oral quinine (10 mg/kg body weight every 8 hours) should be started and continued until 7 days of therapy are completed. Depending on local drug resistance patterns, other oral drugs (sulfadoxine/pyrimethamine, mefloquine, halofantrine) can be added to the regimen in order to reduce the amount of quinine used over time, which, in turn, will reduce the likelihood of quinine-associated side effects. For example, in areas where sulfadoxine/pyrimethamine is effective, after 3 days of quinine therapy, a treatment dose can be given and the quinine discontinued (provided the patient can take oral medications and the parasitemia responded well to the initial quinine treatment). NOTE: Mefloquine should not be given within 12 hours of the last administration of quinine.

Caution: Patients, especially pregnant women, being treated with intravenous quinine or quinidine are at risk of quinine-induced hyperinsulinemic hypoglycemia and should be closely monitored.

Caution: The following ancillary treatments are not effective and in some cases can be harmful and should not be used in the treatment of severe malaria: corticosteroids (e.g., dexamethasone), osmotic/diuretic agents used for treatment of cerebral edema (e.g., mannitol), heparin, adrenalin, and iron chelating drugs (e.g., desferrioxamine B).

SOURCE: World Health Organization (2000a).
NOTE: See Appendix C for alternative regimens.

General Considerations for Malaria Treatment

1. Severe or not?

All patients must be assessed for severe disease and those identified as having severe malaria must immediately be started on appropriate therapy or referred to a facility where that is possible. Danger signs for severe malaria include:

- Inability to take oral medications/fluids;
- Impaired consciousness, unarousable coma;
- Convulsions;
- Severe anemia;
- Organ dysfunction, including renal failure, pulmonary edema, jaundice;
- Hypoglycemia;
- Circulatory collapse and shock;
- Disseminated intravascular coagulation;
- Hyperpyrexia;
- Fluid/electrolyte imbalance; and
- Macroscopic hemoglobinuria.

NOTE: Potential causes of these signs and symptoms other than malaria should also be investigated.

In situations where parasitological diagnosis and quantification are possible, the level of parasitemia can be used as an indication of severity and prognosis. Monitoring parasite density over time is an important aid in patient management and early detection of probable drug resistance or inadequate/ineffective treatment. Among patients with low or no acquired immunity to malaria, parasitemias above 5 percent of infected red blood cells is an indication of severe illness requiring parenteral therapy. Among populations with a high degree of acquired immunity to malaria, parasite loads can be much higher with few symptoms. Observation of schizonts on peripheral blood smears is also an indication of severe illness and of poor prognosis.

2. Plasmodium falciparum or not?

Nonsevere illness presumed to be malaria should, whenever possible, be diagnosed by species. If species-specific diagnosis is not possible, all patients should be treated for *P. falciparum.*

3. Resistant or not?

Because there are no practical bedside tests for drug resistance, all *P. falciparum* infections should be presumed to be resistant if drug resistance is known or believed to be present at high levels in a given area. Determination of risk of drug resistance based solely on prevailing clinical impressions is usually faulty and unreliable. Whenever possible, drug resistance status should be determined by actual assessment using standardized methods. This is usually possible even in a complex emergency. Generally, a treatment failure rate during formal drug efficacy studies of more than 25 percent is used as an indication that alternative treatment should be provided to patients.

In areas where chloroquine-resistant *P. vivax* is common (e.g., parts of Indonesia and Oceania), it should be treated as for *P. falciparum* In areas where chloroquine-resistant *P. vivax* occurs but is uncommon, vivax infections can be initially treated with chloroquine and reassessed for treatment failure at a later date.

4. Concomitant illness?

Malaria is often complicated by concomitant illnesses, such as anemia and malnutrition. This is especially true in displaced populations. Often, the signs and symptoms of malaria can be confused with those of other illnesses (such as pneumonia) and vice versa. This is especially problematic in areas that rely on clinical diagnosis of malaria and other diseases.

careful and attentive nursing to reduce case fatality rates. This care should be available 24 hours a day, 7 days a week. Some general considerations for nursing care are as follows (World Health Organization, 2000a):

- Comatose patients are at risk of aspiration of fluids and must be kept on their sides.
- Patients should be turned frequently to avoid bed sores.
- Hyperthermia (rectal temperature >39°C) should be identified quickly and managed with antipyretics, tepid sponging, and fanning.

Careful monitoring of patients is needed, including their mental status, fluid administration rates, fluid intake and output, glucose, temperature, pulse, respiration, parasite density, and blood pressure.

TREATMENT OF MALARIA DURING PREGNANCY

In populations with little or no immunity, malaria can be a very serious infection, with a high risk of severe maternal morbidity or mortality and fetal loss (Nosten et al., 1991; World Health Organization, 2000a). In populations with high levels of acquired immunity, the primary complications of malaria during pregnancy are maternal anemia and low-birthweight babies, with increased risk primarily seen among women with first or second pregnancies (McGregor, 1984). In either setting, the impact of malaria during pregnancy can be great. Drug resistance, however, has greatly complicated the provision of safe and effective malaria treatment during pregnancy.

The choice of an appropriate first-line treatment for malaria in pregnant women should be based on local drug resistance patterns and the underlying level of immunity of the population. Treatment of otherwise uncomplicated malaria during pregnancy generally follows the recommendations for treatment of uncomplicated malaria in nonpregnant individuals. There are, however, a few drugs that are contraindicated for use during pregnancy and should be avoided (e.g., primaquine, tetracycline, and related drugs).

In many settings, quinine is often the drug of choice for treating symptomatic malaria during pregnancy. While artemisinins have been used successfully and safely during pregnancy (primarily in combination with mefloquine) and may in fact be preferable to quinine (because of a combination of efficacy, ease of administration, and low incidence of side effects,

Use of Artemisinin-Containing Combinations During Pregnancy

CAUTION: Based on limited data, artemisinin + mefloquine combination therapy appears to be safe during the second and third trimesters of pregnancy; its safety in the first semester has not been established (McGready et al., 1998). Animal studies suggest that artemisinin can cause early fetal loss at relatively low doses. Other combinations (artemisinin + sulfadoxine/pyrimethamine or amodiaquine) have not been studied extensively for safety during pregnancy, although based on the record of the components individually, there is currently no reason to suspect they would be harmful. More data are required before a definitive statement on the safety of artemisinin during pregnancy can be made.

especially hypoglycemia) for the treatment of malaria during pregnancy, their safety has not been fully established (McGready et al., 1998). This is especially so for use during the first trimester of pregnancy. Until more experience has been gained with the use of artemisinins (alone or in combination with other drugs), a definitive statement on their safety in pregnancy cannot be made. Nonetheless, artemisinin derivatives, alone or in combination with another safe drug, offer one of the few highly effective treatment options during pregnancy in areas where multidrug-resistant malaria occurs (McGready et al., 1998).

DIAGNOSIS AND TREATMENT OF MALARIA-ASSOCIATED ANEMIA

Anemia is a frequent and clinically important complication of malaria, as it can significantly add to morbidity and mortality in displaced populations. Nevertheless, it is frequently overlooked, especially during complex emergencies. Implementing a systematic assessment for anemia (see Table 6-2), as part of an initial patient evaluation, will likely identify many more patients needing treatment for anemia than would otherwise be identified. Preparations for this increase in patient load associated with anemia should be made in advance. Given the staff and equipment limitations in most emergency situations, many of the options listed in Table 6-2 are not being implemented. Training staff to include pallor as part of their initial examination is an easy first step in addressing this complication. However, it is also important to remember that anemia can be the result of a wide range of infectious and noninfectious causes and that often more than one cause can be identified in a given patient or population.

The single most important component of the management of anemia in areas where malaria poses a significant risk is effective antimalarial treatment. In these areas all anemic patients would likely benefit from effective treatment for malaria, regardless of blood smear status, in addition to whatever anthelminthic, micronutrient, or other ancillary treatment might be appropriate to the setting.

A blood transfusion can be a life-saving intervention, but it can also be unnecessary or even harmful, especially if screening for bloodborne

TABLE 6-2 Some Available Diagnostic Procedures and Tests for Anemia

Test	Sensitivity	Specificity
Clinical diagnosis based on pallor	64% (for Hb <7 g/dl)	64 to 100%
Filter paper and color chart such as WHO Hemoglobin Color Scale[a]	60% (at Hb <10 g/dl) to 90%	60% (at Hb <10 g/dl) to 90%
Copper sulfate method[b]	88%	99%
Sahli Method[c]	85%	85%
Hematocrit	>90%	
Hemoglobinometers such as HemoCue	85 to 100%	94%

[a] The World Health Organization's (WHO) Hemoglobin Color Scale compares the color of a blood spot on filter paper with a standardized color scale.
[b] The copper sulfate method measures the ability of a drop of blood to float or sink in copper sulfate solutions of known specific gravity to determine hemoglobin concentration.

pathogens is not reliable or universally applied (Lackritz, 1998; Obonyo et al., 1998; Kinde-Gazard et al., 2000). Studies have shown that the survival benefit of transfusion is greatest for severely anemic patients with signs of respiratory distress (Lackritz et al., 1992, 1997). This respiratory distress is due to an underlying severe metabolic acidosis (English et al., 1997; World Health Organization, 2000a; Day et al., 2000). Furthermore, severely anemic patients with or without respiratory distress had improved survival only when transfusions were given within the first 24 to 48 hours of admission. Additionally, in one study the presence of malaria parasitemia *after* transfusion negated the hematological benefits of transfusion, suggesting the need for providing severely anemic children with some form of malaria prevention in addition to blood transfusion (Lackritz et al., 1997). Development of guidelines (that are appropriate to the local situation) for the proper use of blood transfusions and training in the recognition of respira-

Comments	References
Training important.	Luby et al. (1995), PATH (1997), Mabeza et al. (2000), Muhe et al. (1998)
Accuracy increases with Hb <9 g/dl.	Stott and Lewis (1995)
More sensitive with Hb <9 g/dl.	PATH (1997)
Special equipment required.	PATH (1997)
Requires centrifuge and electricity for optimum accuracy.	PATH (1997)
Requires relatively expensive equipment and expendable supplies.	PATH (1997)

[c]The Sahli method compares the color of a glass standard to the color of a blood sample after hemoglobin has been converted to acid hematin by the addition of hydrochloric acid.
NOTES: dl = deciliter

tory distress need to be emphasized to ensure optimal management of severe malarial anemia (World Health Organization, 2000a; English et al., 1997).

Nutritional supplementation, especially when combined with effective malaria treatment, can greatly enhance hematological recovery among anemic patients. A strategy worth further investigation is adding post-hospitalization malaria prevention (via drugs or insecticide-treated bed nets) in combination with micronutrient supplementation as a way to further improve hematological status (see also Preventive Use of Antimalarial Drugs, Chapter 7). Some data, however, suggest that concurrent folate supplementation may increase treatment failures of sulfadoxine/pyrimethamine for malaria treatment (van Hensbroek et al., 1995; Shankar, 2000; Bayley and Macreadie, 2002). The appropriate response to these observations is unclear and is being studied. Until more information is available, it would probably be best to withhold folate supplementation, at least temporarily, after treatment with an antifol antimalarial in order to gain maximum benefit from the malaria treatment.

RECOMMENDATIONS

• Identify the differences in levels of transmission and immunity for both the environment from which the displaced population comes and the environment in which it settles to help guide the development of curative and preventive strategies.

• Involve the host government (if functioning) immediately and constructively in discussions about the health needs of the displaced population. Unilateral decisions on the part of relief organizations are unlikely to be welcomed by the host government. The host government may well have pertinent information, advice, and expertise that could be brought to the situation. Discussions should include the consideration of treatment policies, local drug resistance patterns, acceptability, availability, cost, and other operational factors when establishing malaria treatment guidelines.

• Obtain specific local information regarding current drug resistance patterns from standardized drug efficacy trials, the host country's data, and other sources of technical information (such as malaria country profiles from Roll Back Malaria in order to choose the optimal first-line treatment guidelines.

• Use laboratory-based (microscopy) diagnosis whenever feasible.

• Supplement clinical diagnosis (if used) with rapid blood smear surveys to evaluate the reliability of clinical diagnosis on a regular basis.

• Train clinical staff in the recognition and proper treatment of severe malarial disease and important malaria-related complications, such as anemia.

• Establish a referral system to facilitate the transfer of severely ill patients from peripheral health posts to central facilities capable of providing proper management.

• Institute laboratory-based diagnosis for all referral sites to aid in the management of severe disease.

7

Preventive Interventions

The acute emergency phase of a typical complex emergency lasts about four weeks,[1] as relief organizations become better organized and able to meet the needs of the displaced or refugee population, major epidemic illnesses are controlled or prevented, nutritional programs begin to have an effect, the water supply approaches minimal requirements, and shelter is improved. As the situation becomes more stable, public health needs change. Malaria programs need to change too, from emphasizing curative services and reaction to real or potential epidemics to a more sustained control effort. This requires much more emphasis on community involvement in establishing interventions that are cost effective and sustainable.

Appropriate preventive services for malaria control must be defined based on the specifics of the local malaria situation but might include consideration of cost-effective and sustainable vector control strategies (e.g., insecticide-treated nets), prevention of malaria during pregnancy, environmental control, or even prophylaxis of high-risk groups.

---

[1]As described in Chapter 2, there is much variation in the terms used to describe the stages of a complex emergency. Rather than trying to define a specific time period when preventive services are most required, it is more pragmatic to focus on the period of time when the most pressing critical needs are being met in a routine manner, most likely as a result of humanitarian efforts being operationally functional.

PREVENTIVE USE OF ANTIMALARIAL DRUGS

Generally, prophylaxis of large populations is not realistic. Attempts to implement malaria prophylaxis strategies on a large scale have consistently faltered. Noncompliance rates are high, overall cost is high, and long-term sustainability is low. For these reasons mass chemoprophylaxis for malaria control in large populations is not recommended. There are other situations, however, where limited use of malaria prophylaxis is worth considering. Discrete populations, especially groups with little or no immunity to malaria, for which daily or weekly contact with a health care provider is possible may benefit from prophylaxis. Although relatively few evaluations have been done, in either stable or displaced populations, prophylaxis strategies for defined groups such as pregnant women, orphans, unaccompanied minors, or laborers who are housed together for prolonged periods of time could be both effective and manageable.

Preventive Use of Antimalarial Drugs During Pregnancy

Pregnancy is a situation where malaria prevention should be actively encouraged, as pregnant women are at greater risk of malaria infection than nonpregnant women. However, the practical realities mentioned above make such preventive intervention difficult. While chemoprophylaxis during pregnancy has traditionally been the intervention of choice, a relative lack of drugs that are both suitable for prophylaxis and safe during pregnancy as well as poor compliance and widespread drug resistance normally preclude the use of chemoprophylaxis in most areas (Schultz et al., 1994; Steketee, Wirima, and Slutsker, et al., 1996; Robb, 1999). Nonetheless, in areas without chloroquine resistance, weekly prophylaxis with the drug offers a safe and effective method for prevention of placental malaria infection (providing compliance can be maintained at high levels). Mefloquine has been used prophylactically to prevent malaria during pregnancy and has been shown to be both safe and effective (Nosten et al., 1994b), although more recently concerns have been raised about a possible association between mefloquine use during pregnancy and an increased risk of stillbirth (Nosten et al., 1999b).

In areas where chloroquine or mefloquine resistance is common, where mefloquine is not financially viable, or where prophylaxis schemes are unsustainable (which accounts for most malarious areas of the world), alternative strategies to prophylaxis are needed. Often, in these areas and/

or populations the only routinely available strategy, often by default, is one based on prompt diagnosis and effective case management. In some places, because of multidrug resistance and a lack of effective drugs that can be used prophylactically, case management is the only viable strategy, although it is insufficient to eliminate the adverse impact of malaria in pregnancy (Nosten et al., 1991; McGready et al., 1998, 2000).

Among populations in sub-Saharan Africa with a high level of acquired immunity, many malaria infections during pregnancy are asymptomatic (Phillips-Howard, 1999). Additionally, as mentioned previously, most attempts to rely on weekly chemoprophylaxis during pregnancy have met with failure, primarily due to resistance to the drugs most commonly used for prophylaxis (chloroquine) and poor compliance. Therefore, at least in areas of intense stable malaria transmission, neither case management nor weekly chemoprophylaxis can be relied on to adequately protect women and their fetuses from malaria. In such situations, intermittent protective treatment (IPT) with sulfadoxine/pyrimethamine (SP) during the second and third trimesters of pregnancy has been shown to be both an effective and a cost-effective method of preventing malaria-associated maternal anemia and low birth weight (Schultz et al., 1994, 1995; Verhoeff et al., 1997; Parise et al., 1998; Shulman et al., 1999). IPT differs from chemoprophylaxis in that chemoprophylaxis refers to frequent use of a drug (either daily or weekly, depending on the nature of the drug) in order to prevent illness. IPT refers to intermittent treatment doses of a drug given presumptively (i.e., not based on presence of illness or demonstrated malaria infection) on a less-frequent basis (such as monthly or even less often). The purpose is to periodically clear existing infections and, depending on the nature of the drug, provide a period of lingering protection from illness. The latter effect is achieved when using drugs for IPT, such as SP, that have long half-lives (essentially, the period of time needed for the blood concentration to be reduced by half). After a drug is given, blood drug levels peak and then diminish over time as the drug is eliminated from the body: as long as the drug blood level remains above the minimum required to inhibit parasite growth, the patient should be protected from malarial illness.

Because of the opportunity to link this strategy with antenatal care visits, this approach offers an implementable and sustainable intervention. Various limitations, however, argue against the use of such a strategy in many areas. Resistance to SP is prevalent in South America and Asia and is becoming a serious concern in sub-Saharan Africa. Other antimalarial drugs (mefloquine monotherapy, combination therapy including an artemisinin compound, or other drugs) have not been studied as part of an IPT strategy but may be an option in areas where they are effective for routine treatment of uncomplicated malaria. Among nonimmune populations and/or in areas with low malaria transmission rates, the relative infrequency of infection, the high likelihood that such an infection would be symptomatic, and the real risk that a mild infection could rapidly become severe might decrease the usefulness or effectiveness of an IPT approach. There is a small amount of data that suggest *P. vivax* infections also place pregnant women at risk of anemia and their babies at risk of low birth weight (Nosten et al., 1999a).

HIV Infection and Malaria During Pregnancy

As mentioned previously, later pregnancies (third or more) appear to be at as great a risk of producing low-birthweight babies as first and second pregnancies among women who are HIV (human immunodeficiency virus) seropositive (Steketee et al., 1996b). HIV infection also appears to reduce the protective effect of intermittent antimalarial therapy. Populations with relatively high HIV seroprevalence (>15 percent) have been shown to achieve a high degree of protection against malaria when IPT is given on a monthly basis (Parise et al., 1998).

Prophylaxis of Other High-Risk Populations

Anemic children (especially those who received blood transfusions because of severe anemia), severely malnourished individuals receiving therapeutic feeding, and nonimmune populations newly exposed to malaria transmission would likely benefit from preventive use of antimalarial drugs. This could be accomplished either through routine chemoprophylaxis or by using a system of regular presumptive treatment along the lines of IPT during pregnancy. For example, one study in Africa of presumptive treatment for malaria at the time of routine infant vaccinations reduced the rates of both clinical malaria and severe anemia compared to a placebo treatment (Schellenberg et al., 2001). Prophylaxis or presumptive therapy might also be advisable for severely malnourished individuals. Therapeutic feeding of starved individuals has been shown to reactivate preexisting, but quiescent, malaria infections, with potentially severe consequences (Murray et al., 1976, 1978). A short period of prophylaxis or presumptive treatment during nutritional rehabilitation might prevent these recrudescent infections. Ideally, prevention should include more than a single approach. For example, other measures, such as insecticide-treated bed nets, would be appropriate preventive strategies in many situations.

Other Prevention Issues

A number of intervention studies have investigated the contribution of specific nutrients to exacerbation or prevention of malaria. Parenteral iron supplementation during pregnancy has been shown to increase the risk of malaria infection among primigravidae, whereas oral supplementation of multigravidae did not (Oppenheimer et al., 1986b; Menendez et al., 1994). A clinical trial that provided iron supplementation (with and without malaria prophylaxis) to a population of children less than 1 year old who were exposed to intense perennial malaria transmission was effective at preventing severe anemia and clinical malaria (Menendez et al., 1997). In another study, zinc supplementation reduced clinic attendance due to malaria and dramatically reduced high-density malaria infections (Shankar et al., 2000). Other nutrients that may be important in reducing malaria morbidity or mortality include vitamins A and C, riboflavin, betacarotene, and various antioxidants (Shankar, 2000).

Provision of a program of nutritional supplementation to a displaced population, while difficult, is not impossible. In a study of Burundian refugees in Tanzania, supplementation of moderately anemic children with varying combinations of iron, folic acid, vitamins A and C, and monthly presumptive malaria treatment was achieved using a cadre of home health visitors, resulting in substantial hematological recovery and improvement in iron stores (Tomashek et al., 2001).

INSECTICIDE-TREATED BED NETS

Insecticide-treated nets (ITNs) impregnated with inexpensive and long-lasting pyrethroids have been shown to reduce human-vector contact, inoculation of humans with sporozoites, clinical episodes of fever, high-density parasitemia, malaria-attributed mortality, and overall mortality (Bermejo and Veeken, 1992; Choi et al., 1995; D'Alessandro et al., 1995; Lengeler, 1998). Reviews of published reports suggest that the overall protective efficacy of ITNs for mortality in children less than 5 years old was about 18 percent and against mild malaria episodes 39 to 48 percent (Lengeler, 1998). ITN usage was also associated with higher-packed cell volumes in children. There was also a trend for greater protective efficacy in areas with low-to-medium transmission compared to high transmission.

ITNs have been used for malaria control in displaced populations with success in some settings. In Nepal a combination of ITNs and active case detection and treatment reduced the incidence of malaria from approximately 22 cases per 10,000 persons per day to 0.2 cases (Martin et al., 1994). In Thailand, ITNs reduced *P. falciparum* infections and episodes of clinical malaria among displaced school-aged children and reduced the incidence of malaria-associated anemia in displaced pregnant women (Dolan et al., 1993; Luxemberger et al., 1994). ITNs were also shown to produce a modest reduction in cumulative infection rates of migrant workers in eastern Thailand (Kamol-Ratanakul and Prasittisuk, 1992). ITN programs for Afghan refugees in Pakistan have also met with considerable success (Rowland et al., 1996; Rowland, 1999).

Bed nets are easily installed over beds or floor mats, can be readily moved, protect one or more persons (depending on users' ages and the sizes of the nets available), provide some warmth and enhanced privacy at night, are generally affordable, and can last for years with proper care. The process of impregnating and hanging the nets is not complicated. Studies have clearly demonstrated that motivated community members can be taught to use bed nets properly and to do the impregnation, drying, hanging, and maintenance with only modest assistance from local governmental health staff.

Depending on seasonality of malaria transmission and the frequency of washing, bed nets may require retreatment as often as twice per year or more frequently (World Health Organization, 1997c). Low retreatment rates of nets have frequently been identified as an important obstacle to implementing an effective ITN program (Cham et al., 1997; Curtis and Mnzava, 2000). "Permanently" treated nets (also known as wash-durable or long-lasting insecticide-treated nets) have been developed and are being evaluated under field conditions (Guillet et al., 2001). While use of these nets may increase initial program costs, the elimination of the need for retreatment may make them more effective over the life of the net.

If ITNs are widely distributed and used in a community, infective vector density should be reduced, resulting in decreased vector-human contact, lowered malaria transmission, and decreased morbidity and mortality. These effects can occur even when ITNs are torn and benefit extends to nonnet users in the same house (Lindsay et al., 1991). At higher levels of coverage, protection extends even to non-users of ITNs living in nearby houses (Howard et al., 2000). Recent data from an area of intense transmission suggest that coverage needs to be at least 50 to 60 percent in order to achieve these community benefits (W. Hawley, Centers for Disease Control and Prevention, personal communication, 2002). In fact, recent studies suggest that the effectiveness of insecticide-treated nets is due primarily to the action of the insecticide and the extent of coverage, while the physical barrier effect is of minimal importance (Hawley et al., in press). For this reason, if ITNs are to be used, rapid implementation aimed at achieving high coverage should be stressed to obtain maximal benefits from the program. ITN programs that achieve low coverage rates or fail to treat (or retreat) nets appropriately with insecticide are likely to accomplish little more than the wasting of valuable resources (Hawley et al., in press).

Insecticide-Treated Curtains

Insecticide-treated curtains (ITCs) have been shown to reduce human-vector contact and to reduce morbidity and mortality due to malaria (Cuzin-Ouattara et al., 1999; Habluetzel et al., 1997, 1999). In certain circumstances ITCs could play an important role, especially where refugee housing consists of small houses with one room, one door, and one or no windows. In such cases, ITNs would hinder movement around and use of the room, whereas curtains would be out of the way yet serve essentially the same purpose.

Economic Feasibility

The economic feasibility of using ITNs as an intervention has been examined in a number of settings. The cost to distribute ITNs to an entire camp population of displaced Karen in Thailand was examined (Luxemberger et al., 1994). The number of malaria treatments for *P. falciparum* that would be avoided by ITN use was estimated to be 310 to 1,748. (The cost to treat this number of cases of malaria would be $744 to $4,195.) Although this may have been a cost-effective intervention over the course of a number of years, the life span of the net, generally only about a year in that environment, was judged to be the most important obstacle.

In terms of the cost to the community itself, an investment in a successful ITN intervention in both Malawi and Cameroon would be outweighed by the savings associated with decreased morbidity and decreased mortality due to caring for sick individuals (Brinkmann and Brinkmann, 1995). In the Gambia the estimated cost of death averted by a successful ITN intervention was $600, a cost thought to compare favorably with other interventions, such as measles vaccination and oral rehydration solutions (D'Alessandro et al., 1995).

ITN use also compared favorably to other vector control methods. In the Solomon Islands the per-capita cost of an ITN program was $1.97 compared with a per-capita program cost of $4.37 for indoor residual spraying with dichlorodiphenyltrichloroethane (DDT); efficacy data were not available (Kere and Kere, 1992). In South Africa, ITN use, while more effective in terms of reducing malaria cases, was found to be more expensive than residual house spraying (Goodman et al., 2001). However, the price per net used in this analysis was substantially higher than current market prices, and, assuming more typical net prices, the cost of using ITNs would have been lower than using residual spraying. Furthermore, by including costs saved through decreased treatment of malaria cases, ITNs would have resulted in a net savings. Using established guidelines, both ITN programs and residual spray programs would be considered cost effective and attractive health investments (cost per disability-adjusted life year averted was less than $150; Goodman et al., 1999).

The cost of an ITN program will depend on bed net size, model, type, quality of material, and country (MacCormack et al., 1989). Prices for both nets and insecticides vary by country and product. Wholesale net prices are currently under $4 and in some areas even less (Goodman et al., 2001). Similarly, costs for insecticides vary widely but are generally low.

OTHER PERSONAL PROTECTION MEASURES

People can help protect themselves from acquiring malaria (or other vectorborne diseases) by using simple measures that decrease the likelihood of coming into contact with vectors. Through a basic understanding of the vector's habits, especially the time of day it most likely feeds, people can modify their behavior and/or activity patterns to decrease their exposure. For example, many malaria vectors are particularly active from late dusk to dawn; if people use repellents on their exposed skin and clothes, wear long pants, long-sleeved shirts, and a hat, and stay indoors behind screened entries, their risk of exposure to disease-carrying vectors will be greatly reduced. Obviously, in many situations associated with rapid or unplanned migration, these measures are unlikely, impractical, or impossible and, even under optimal conditions, would be difficult to implement and sustain. These measures may be beneficial on an individual level, but on a population basis they would probably have, at best, only a limited effect on malaria morbidity.

Repellents

Permethrin, a synthetic pyrethroid, can be used to impregnate clothing to repel insects. While it is very effective in preventing insects from biting through impregnated clothing, it offers minimal protection to exposed skin. Permethrin-impregnated clothing can be washed a number of times and still retain sufficient material to repel insects. This approach has been used effectively among some Afghan refugees in Pakistan by impregnating blankets or chaddars, a traditional wrap worn by Afghan women and used by both men and women as a sheet at night (Rowland et al., 1999; Rowland, 2001). The cost of treating chaddars was estimated to be $0.17 per person. Since chaddars were already used by these communities, this strategy avoided the additional cost of net purchase (Rowland et al., 1999).

DEET (N,N-diethyl-m-toluamide) is a repellent used on exposed skin. It is effective for a number of hours, but perspiration reduces its effectiveness. Soap containing a combination of DEET and permethrin has been evaluated in a number of settings, none involving complex emergencies (Kroeger et al., 1997). Although protective efficacy was generally high when soap was used, motivation for continued use over time was low, and factors such as activity level and sweating adversely affected its impact. Since distribution of soap has other health benefits, including reduction of diarrheal disease, and is a frequent inclusion in refugee provisions, even a small added benefit might be worth the incremental expense of distributing repellent soaps (Peterson et al., 1998). However, soap distribution in general remains inadequate in most situations of displacement. In Peru and Ecuador in 1997, soap distribution was estimated to cost $4.60 per person per year (Kroeger et al., 1997).

VECTOR CONTROL USING INSECTICIDES

Role of Vector Control in Emergencies

The role of insecticidal vector control in an emergency setting will depend, to a great extent, on the local epidemiology of malaria, the feeding and resting behavior of the major mosquito vectors, and the capacity of relief organizations to mount and sustain vector control activities. A knowledgeable entomologist should be consulted regarding the appropriateness of vector control using insecticides, which insecticide(s) to use for a given intervention and area, and proper use and application of insecticides.

The two principal methods of using insecticides for vector control are larvaciding and adulticiding. Larvaciding is the control of mosquito breeding with insecticides. This form of control is most effective when only a few discrete breeding sites are responsible for the majority of the transmission but can become impossible if breeding sites are poorly defined or numerous. For example, *An. gambiae* (an important malaria vector in most areas of sub-Saharan Africa) frequently breed in almost any groundwater, from hoofprints to flooded rice fields. The cost is proportional to the area of water to be treated, so the method may not be economical except where there are high-density larval populations.

Adulticiding (using insecticides to kill adult mosquitoes) is technically less demanding, requiring more training but less skill. It is effective against vectors that rest on the walls of houses either before or after taking blood. The cost is proportional to the number of houses treated. Historically, in most circumstances adulticiding proved to be more useful than larvaciding and should be used preferentially unless it can be proven that larvicidal application is practical and effective, such as might occur when the vector bites outside houses and breeding sites are few and well defined.

Adulticiding can be accomplished with residual or space spraying. Residual spraying involves the application of insecticides to the inside walls of a building, tent, or other shelter. It is most effective against mosquito vectors that both bite and rest indoors. Mosquitoes that immediately leave the structure after feeding are obviously not exposed to the insecticide. Space spraying is aimed primarily at killing flying mosquitoes and is generally a far less efficient and cost-effective method of mosquito control. It has been used in epidemic situations in order to get a rapid decrease in adult mosquito populations and as a highly visible intervention.

ITNS OR RESIDUAL SPRAYING IN REFUGEE SETTINGS?

Studies have shown that in most settings ITNs and residual spraying programs have approximately the same level of efficacy and cost effectiveness for preventing malaria (Goodman et al., 1999; Curtis and Mnzava, 2000). Comparisons between programs (or studies) using either ITNs or residual spraying do not give a clear answer in terms of cost. In some settings nets were less expensive; in others spray programs were less expensive. Therefore, the decision to opt for one over the other for malaria control for a displaced population revolves around local logistical constraints. Provided that either could be used effectively against locally prevalent malaria vectors, they each have their advantages and disadvantages.

It is important to remember that net distribution will not ensure that the nets will be kept, will be used properly, or that the most vulnerable members of households will benefit from their use. Among displaced populations, ITNs can be viewed as a valuable commodity to be traded for other desired goods, such as food items, or sold for cash. In camps in western Tanzania, almost 50 percent of nets distributed to Burundian refugees were missing less than 3 months later; in a second camp only about 15 percent of nets remained 1.5 years after original distribution (International Rescue Committee, unpublished data, 1997). This is a problem that may diminish over time as communities become more stable and the benefits of net use are more widely appreciated, but trading or selling nets rather than using them can clearly compromise the public health impact of an ITN program (Curtis and Mnzava, 2000; Rowland, 2001).

ITN use presumes that a displaced population has shelter that can accommodate a net. While nets can be made to fit into very small shelters, those commercially available in large quantities are typically too large to fit in many shelters commonly found in refugee camps, especially early in an emergency phase.

Successful ITN use is highly dependent on community acceptance and participation. Not only does the community need to use the nets, its residents must adhere to reimpregnation schedules for optimal effect. Among some stable populations, nets are often used exclusively by the male head of household, leaving the more vulnerable children unprotected (Makemba et al., 1995; Van Bortel et al., 1996).

In comparison, residual spraying requires only passive community participation. Spray teams can rapidly move through a settlement and achieve complete coverage in a short period of time. Residual spraying does not require any specific behavioral change on the part of household members (Rowland, 1999). However, some shelter types would not be amenable to residual spraying; insecticides do not stick well to plastic sheeting, although residual spraying of cotton and canvas tents was effective for refugee populations in Pakistan (Hewitt et al., 1995). Studies are under way to develop methods to impregnate shelter materials, such as plastic and canvas sheeting, and blankets (Rowland, 2001; World Health Organization, 2001a).

Even when ITNs are preferable, it may take time and stability to successfully implement an ITN program. Adequate time and effort should be placed on designing the most appropriate community education program in order to teach the proper use of nets and to highlight vulnerable populations who most need this protection. In such situations a residual spray campaign could be used early in a complex emergency for rapid coverage, and then, as the situation stabilizes, there would be a transition to an ITN strategy. In the Tanzanian camps mentioned previously, the nongovernmental organization on the scene stopped campwide ITN distribution in favor of a twice-yearly residual spraying campaign, while community health workers attempted to improve ITN use through health education.

ENVIRONMENTAL AND BIOLOGICAL VECTOR CONTROL

When vector breeding sites are few in number and easily identified, environmental or biological control may be a viable option. Environmental management strategies include such activities as draining or filling in pools of water, modifying the boundaries of rivers or other water drainage systems, and applying materials to open water, such as oil or styrofoam beads, to disrupt larval development. Biological control strategies, including use of bacteria (such as *Bacillus thuringiensis* subsp. *israelensis*, or *Bti*) or larvivorous fish, have also been used with other control measures and with variable levels of success (Karch et al., 1992; Romi et al., 1993, World Health Organization, 1999a; Kaneko et al., 2000). Data that prove the effectiveness of some commonly recommended environmental control measures against malaria, such as cutting or clearing grass from around dwellings, are lacking. If the situation permits, the location of settlement areas for displaced populations should be chosen or reviewed with attention to the potential risk for vectorborne disease. Similarly, planning for developmental projects should include consideration of the impact on vector breeding sites (World Health Organization, 1998).

RECOMMENDATIONS

• Review supply management procedures and ensure a reliable source of antimalarial drugs, nets or curtains (if used), and insecticides.

- Ensure prompt, safe, and effective case management of malaria for all pregnant women.
- Establish intermittent protective treatment for pregnant women in areas with high malaria transmission.
- Seek guidance from an experienced medical entomologist to identify and implement appropriate cost-effective vector control strategies.
- Consider initial use of a residual spray program, even if insecticide-treated nets are ultimately used, to achieve rapid protection and to afford sufficient time to develop and implement a sustainable net program.
- Consider ways to integrate malaria prevention for children and pregnant women with nutritional support activities and/or antenatal care.
- Design an appropriate community education program to teach proper use of nets and to highlight vulnerable populations who most need this protection (if a net program is deemed the best approach to use).
- If insecticide-treated nets are to be used, the rapid attainment of high coverage (>50 percent of households) should be stressed. Reconsider using nets if it is unlikely that high coverage rates can be attained (in such cases, residual spraying may be a more cost-effective approach).

Malaria Prevention Interventions: Key Points

- Malaria control must rapidly evolve from simple provision of curative services to development of a more sustainable control program that includes preventive interventions.
- Preventive services should be tailored to the specific situation and may include a variety of approaches, such as use of insecticide-treated materials or prevention of malaria during pregnancy using intermittent protective treatment.
- Vector control strategies should be formulated on information regarding the local epidemiology of malaria, the feeding and resting behavior of the principal mosquito vectors, and the ability of relief organizations to mount and sustain vector control activities.
- There is an increasing body of evidence pointing to interactions between malaria, anemia, and malnutrition. As evidence accumulates, it may become important to integrate malaria prevention activities with nutritional support activities.

8

Community Involvement in Malaria Control and Prevention

Malaria prevention must go hand in hand with community participation. Unless individuals in communities see the merits of preventing the illness, even the best-designed prevention strategies might not be used. It is necessary to understand how a community perceives febrile illness, the importance placed on it in people's belief systems regarding illness in general, and what existing behaviors are practiced that can either complement or hinder preventive measures.

The use of preventive measures will be affected by two things: how affected communities define their priorities regarding health and illness and the degree to which individuals think they can personally control or prevent illness. No matter how sound a preventive approach might be, if individuals do not see the merits of a particular approach or if competing needs are prioritized higher, the preventive approaches will fail to some degree. A key question is what personal protection measures are acceptable to the population at risk: What is their history in using preventive measures? Are there any cultural taboos or fears associated with preventive measures? For example, if pregnant women are concerned about using antimalarial drugs during pregnancy, it would be necessary to offer comprehensive health education about malaria risks during pregnancy prior to implementing protective intermittent treatment programs. If malaria (or febrile illness in general) is perceived as an illness for which personal actions cannot modify the acquisition or course of the illness, preventive behaviors would probably not be viewed as important.

In many situations involving displaced populations, resource limitations may restrict the types of preventive services that can be offered or to which subpopulations such services could be offered. Ideally, scarce resources should be applied first to those groups at greatest risk. However, this leads to the question of what constitutes vulnerability and whose definition is used when making programmatic decisions about resources. Nongovernmental organizations (NGOs) and communities might not agree on who is most vulnerable. For example, a health-related NGO might label children under 5 years of age and pregnant women as the most vulnerable, whereas communities might identify displaced individuals working in jobs with humanitarian agencies as the most vulnerable. Time lost from work because of malaria would be seen as a threat to these scarce jobs, which are often seen as "prime positions" in terms of receiving additional rations or other advantages.

DEFINITION OF VULNERABILITY

It becomes necessary early in an emergency to determine how a community defines "vulnerability"—that is, who within a population is most in need of preventive measures. Studies of famine and food distribution in complex emergencies show that vulnerability is a poorly understood concept (Jaspers and Shoham, 1999; Webb and Harinarayan, 1999). In addition to physiological parameters of vulnerability (such as age and parity for malaria), vulnerability is partly determined by social, political, and economic factors. The dynamics of vulnerability that mitigate a crisis and lessen the impact for some people but not others are not well understood. In planning malaria prevention programs, nontraditional segments of the potential population at risk in a complex emergency should also be considered as vulnerable. For example, are there any marginalized subgroups for whom participation in preventive programs (such as an insecticide-treated net reimpregnation program) might not be feasible due to security concerns? Other socially vulnerable groups might include self-settled rural refugees or internally displaced persons, elderly persons, disabled persons, or even female-headed households. The implications for their access to both malaria prevention and management have not been given adequate attention in complex emergencies. Also, there is limited information on socioeconomic factors that influence the prevalence of malaria. What is known is based on nonemergency situations in Africa (Guiguemde et al., 1994; Koram et al., 1995a, 1995b).

BEHAVIORS AND RISK

Consideration should also be given to behaviors that might place a displaced population at risk for malaria. Does labor migration occur? If so, where? What are the hours of potential exposure? As mentioned in Chapter 1, one risk factor for displaced populations is no or poor housing. Particularly in the early stages of a complex emergency, people might be housed in tents or under plastic sheeting tarpaulins, both of which are incompatible with the proper hanging of standard insecticide-treated bed nets or with residual spraying. Another risk factor, depending on the biting preferences of the vector, might be the presence of livestock.

In determining the merits of using preventive measures, such as insecticide-treated materials, questions should be raised about the social market value of such measures. If packages of rations do not contain items that are accepted and valued, those rations might well be sold or traded for other things perceived as being more valuable. For example, mosquito nets might be traded for blankets or items of food that are more highly desired by refugees. In planning prevention programs it is also important to determine who makes financial decisions for households, to identify to whom the rations are distributed, and to clarify who is considered most vulnerable and in need of preventive measures. It is not a certainty that children under age 5 or pregnant women will be allowed to sleep under a mosquito net, particularly if there is only one net in the household. Designing preventive approaches for displaced populations takes creative thought, given the constraints of situations where people have little control over where they live or the types of shelter available to them.

HUMAN BEHAVIOR AND MALARIA CONTROL: SOCIOCULTURAL CONSIDERATIONS

An important element to any aspect of malaria control is human behavior—an understanding of what people perceive as the cause of malaria, the extent to which they believe they can prevent and/or treat malaria, and their acceptance and usage of malaria control interventions. These are determining factors in the success or failure of a malaria control program. Influences from the larger context (political, social, cultural, environmental, and economic) in which people live their daily lives affect personal choices and may influence whether a control program is sustainable. For example, access to health care and the ability to buy antimalarial drugs may be predicated on several things, such as personal knowledge about malaria, extent of poverty, seasonal variations in income, or even whether or not a functional road or transportation system exists. In complex emergencies, contextual factors often become more complicated—for example, expectations of what constitutes "appropriate" malaria treatment from the perspective of the displaced population may contrast with the type of treatment offered at the refugee camp.

Too often, malaria control activities are designed with little understanding of the cultural context in which they are supposed to operate. Relief agency staff become frustrated and angry that a seemingly good and logical proposal has failed to capture the interests of the at-risk populations for which it was designed. Additionally, decisions about whether to take action and which actions to take are often based on sociopolitical factors and not necessarily scientific data. These influences must be considered as well when attempting to engage agencies and at-risk populations in malaria control activities.

Perceptions of Febrile Illness

Understanding how febrile illness in general is perceived is the first step in understanding how individuals conceive of malaria as a disease entity. What is defined and understood as "malaria" from a biomedical perspective may or may not match the local understanding of the illness. Perceived etiology of fever (specifically, "malaria fever") will determine, in part, treatment-seeking behavior (Williams et al., 1999).

Ethnographic work from the coastal areas of Tanzania is a good example of the impact of people's perceptions of illness (Winch et al., 1996; Winch, 1999). In this setting, routine or mild fever is grouped five ways: "malaria fever" (*homa ya malaria*, in KiSwahili), fever due to personal problems, periodic fevers, ordinary fever, and fever from boils. Including "malaria fever" in this group indicates that it is not perceived as a serious illness, which could have implications for how rapidly people seek treatment as well as the source of treatment. *Homa ya malaria* is associated with the use of formal health care services. Illnesses that have symptoms associated with severe malaria are grouped with severe fevers or illnesses associated with sorcery or witchcraft, which are best treated by traditional practitioners. There is also a separate classification of a childhood illness (*degedege*) whose symptoms were compatible with severe malaria (including cerebral malaria) but were not linked with *homa ya malaria*. Perceived to be a spiritual illness, it is thought to be unrelated to malaria in children; thus, the importance of malaria as a potentially fatal disease in children was underestimated in the local population. Local interpretations of febrile illnesses are necessary in order to interpret how, why, when, and from whom people seek medical treatment. It is also important to understand how similar the displaced population is from the host population, particularly if both groups are receiving care from the same facilities.

Treatment-Seeking Behaviors

In addition to the perceived etiology of an illness, there are other factors that will determine treatment-seeking behaviors for malaria. Issues important to understanding treatment seeking include the type(s) of treatment chosen and the timing and sequencing of the treatment. People often choose multiple sources of treatment, both traditional and Western. Antimalarials and other drugs used to treat malaria illness (e.g., antipyretics, antibiotics) are often obtained outside formal health care services (Foster, 1995; McCombie, 1996). Although treatment-seeking studies generally discuss delays in seeking treatment in terms of the time lapse between onset of symptoms and a person seeking treatment at a health care facility, self-treatment for malaria occurs frequently and this may be the first type of treatment sought (McCombie, 1996).

There is almost no documented information about the malaria treatment-seeking practices of displaced populations. If refugees are residing in a camp setting, the distance from the residential units to the health care facilities might be a limiting factor, particularly during nighttime hours. Security issues (e.g., the ability to move freely around the area of refuge without being hassled, fear of rape, accessibility of the settlement area to outsiders) and the availability of communication and transportation between residential areas and health care facilities may delay treatment seeking from established health care facilities. Conversely, if refugees are situated in "open" camps/settlements (camps that permit movement of the displaced population out of the identified area of refuge) or if refugees are self-settled, people may choose to use the health care services provided to the host population.

As emergencies stabilize and periods of displacement become longer in duration, communities attempt to re-create their formal patterns of social organization and informal social structures begin to resemble the preflight period, given the constraints of refuge. In some communities, nonofficial sources of health care, such as traditional healers (herbalists, spiritual healers, bush doctors, etc.), may have been the preferred source of illness treatment during the predisplacement periods. Once "settled" in the area of refuge, members of the community may seek out these healers to treat malaria-like illnesses. Some NGOs have been sensitive to the role that alternative healers have traditionally played in some communities and have incorporated traditional patterns of healing into the services offered by health care facilities. In the Thai/Cambodian camps in the 1980s, traditional healers known as the *Kru Khmer* came to the pediatric inpatient facility on a regular basis to make clinical rounds with the health care staff. The *Kru Khmer* lent support to clinical decisions made by the staff, and families and community leaders were encouraged by the positive recognition of an important element of their culture.

Treatment decisions might also be affected by the choice of drugs used for first-line therapy. In refugee camps in western Tanzania in 1998, Burundian refugees were dismayed by the use of chloroquine as the official first-line therapy, as they had previously used sulfadoxine/pyrimethamine, with better clinical results than when they were treated with chloroquine. Treatment decisions of the host community may also be influenced by case management policies for the displaced population. If members of the host community determine that the displaced community is receiving better care or a more effective drug for malaria, the host community might also try to receive health care services from the humanitarian relief agencies. This could have serious personnel and financial implications for the relief agencies. And perceptions about preferential treatment for the displaced population can lead to feelings of resentment and/or hostility by the host population.

Depending on how quickly markets can be established in the area of refuge (if allowed at all) and the financial resources of those displaced, self-medication with purchased drugs may be common. The availability of antimalarial drugs at health care facilities might also play a role in where people obtain care. If nongovernmental facilities regularly run out of anti-malarial drugs, local markets might play a bigger role in treatment of the disease.

Interactions with the staff of a health care facility may affect treatment choices. In nonemergency contexts, parents of ill children in Africa were reluctant to discuss self-treatment, particularly when employing a traditional healer, for fear of disapproval from health care workers (Williams et al., 1999). A lack of respect toward patients in general from health care workers in Africa has also been noted (van der Geest, 1997). If health care workers are primarily international staff or even national staff from a different cultural background than the affected population, this might diminish the use of health care facilities. How the displaced population perceives the health care workers available to them in a complex emergency is unknown. Gratitude for care received may be an overriding factor, but without documentation of the dynamics between humanitarian relief workers and displaced persons, one can only speculate.

Need for Information on the Sociocultural Aspects of Complex Emergencies

Historically, those involved with health care issues in complex emergencies have given little attention to the sociocultural dimensions or to the wider global context within which complex emergencies develop. Given the complexities of providing essential health care services to displaced populations, particularly in the beginning stages of an emergency, this is understandable. The skills required to gather the types of sociocultural information that could assist in programmatic and policy planning and implementation are not generally found in humanitarian relief agencies. However, this may be a shortsighted view as valuable resources (both financial and human) can be wasted in planning programs to modify behaviors that are not clearly understood or that are based on false assumptions of why people behave in a certain manner.

One approach to address this gap would be for humanitarian organizations to work closely with social scientists, such as medical anthropologists, whose applied training reflects the perspectives of both biomedicine and social science (Williams and Bloland, 2001). There may be social scientists in the displaced population who could work jointly with the humanitarian relief agencies to define the most critical sociocultural questions and identify the most appropriate way to gather and analyze such data.

Acknowledging the situational constraints of complex emergencies (i.e., the need for urgent decision making, the volume of work required to maintain day-to-day operations, limited budgets, and the fluid nature of an emergency), rapid assessments may be the most practical means of gathering data to inform programs, particularly in the early stages of an emergency. Rapid assessments (also called rapid ethnographic assessments, participatory rural appraisals, rapid community assessments, or rapid assessment procedures) refer to individual and group-based ethnographic methods to gather cultural, social, economic, and behavioral data in a rapid fashion (Chambers, 1992; Beebe, 1995; Cornwall and Jewkes, 1995; David et al., 1998; Nichter, 1999). A key component of rapid appraisals is the inclusion of the affected population in all stages of the work, from data collection through analysis. The data obtained reflect the viewpoint of the displaced community, as opposed to the perspective of humanitarian workers or agencies.[1] Also, rapid appraisals often combine qualitative and quantitative approaches, which is particularly useful in addressing epidemiological problems. The following are some examples of questions that could guide the gathering of baseline data for programmatic planning of malaria control:

1. Baseline demographics
- Ethnic and geographical background of displaced population, including subgroups.
- Types of family or household structures: identification of head of household, numbers and types of groups perceived to be vulnerable.
- Religious or cultural practices.
- Community leaders, both formal and informal.
- Degree of social organization currently existing in the displaced population. How different is it from the predisplacement social organization?

2. Perception of illness and treatment-seeking practices
- How is febrile illness understood, particularly in relation to the biomedical conceptualization of malaria?
- What local terms are used to describe febrile illness and malaria?
- How does the community define vulnerability in terms of malaria?
- What influences people to seek treatment? Where, when, how, and by whom is treatment sought? Are there differences by age groups?
- What is the degree of self-treatment? What does it consist of?
- Are there any political, economic, or structural constraints to seeking care?

---

[1]The Center for Refugee and Disaster Studies at the Johns Hopkins University School of Public Health has developed a guide specifically geared toward understanding the perceived needs of refugees and internally displaced persons and is a good reference for fieldwork (Weiss and Bolton, 2000). Available at: <*http://www.jhsph.edu/refugee/images/tqr_a_docs/ tg_introduction.pdf*>.

- How does the malaria treatment offered to the displaced population differ from their home experience?
- What are the perceptions of safety and effectiveness of the antimalarial drugs?

3. Prevention

- What prevention measures are acceptable to the affected population?
- What prevention measures are unacceptable and why?
- What is the social market value of insecticide-treated materials or antimalarial drugs?
- What behaviors, such as labor migration, increase the risk of acquiring malaria?

4. Implementing malaria control

- What is the community's previous experience with malaria control programs?
- What are the priorities for malaria control, as defined by the affected community? How do those priorities differ from those of the relief agencies?
- What possible constraints are there to implementing malaria control (population- or agency-based, financial, political)?
- What would be attractive incentives to encourage and support the displaced population to engage in malaria control activities?

RECOMMENDATIONS

- Identify the most vulnerable populations: pregnant women, children under age 5, and sociopolitical groups that might not be able to access care.
- Identify key members of the affected community to work with representatives from relief agencies.
- Examine sociopolitical influences that might affect the acceptability and use of malaria control strategies.
- Collaborate with applied social scientists to better understand the factors that influence treatment-seeking behaviors by the affected populations.

Role of Community Participation in Malaria Prevention and Control: Key Points

- Community participation (reflecting both understanding and acceptability of interventions) should be an essential element in both malaria prevention and control.
- The sociocultural context surrounding displacement situations needs to be considered when designing malaria control interventions.
- Treatment-seeking behaviors are complex and poorly understood in the context of complex emergencies.

9

Special Studies and Operational Research

In some situations, special studies might be required to more accurately estimate the prevalence or incidence of malaria-associated illness, to evaluate the efficacy of malaria therapy, to determine the principle malaria vectors in the area, or to test new interventions or monitor the effectiveness of existing ones. These operational research issues are necessary in order to make sound programmatic decisions. However, there is a sensitivity about the use of the term "research," even though these research issues are operationally oriented activities.

IS RESEARCH APPROPRIATE AND FEASIBLE IN EMERGENCY SETTINGS?

What Are the Best Practices?

Historically, there has been resistance to conducting research during complex emergencies, particularly during the acute phases of an emergency. The concern was that it is unethical to impose the burden of research on vulnerable populations that are traumatized, frequently in ill health, and attempting to survive in new surroundings. Slowly, this sentiment has been shifting toward the recognition that not only is research needed but that it is unethical to continue to practice public health measures that may or may not reflect "best practices" (Burkle, 1999; Waldman and Martone, 1999; Banatvala and Zwi, 2000; Brundtland, 2000; McClelland et al.,

103

2000; Ezard, 2001a).   However, what constitutes best practices in the context of an emergency is often not known, as the base of applied research in this area is limited (Burkle, 1999). Best practices have been based mostly on summaries of personal and/or organizational experiences, lacking theoretical perspectives and rigorous application of standard clinical, epidemiological, or other scientific methodologies needed to answer research or programmatic questions (Waldman and Williams, 2001). Little research has been documented, as evidenced by a small inventory of health research in emergencies (World Health Organization, 1999b). But initiating research and monitoring and evaluating ongoing malaria control activities are necessary to improve humanitarian relief practices (Dick and Simmonds, 1983; Walkup, 1997; Banatvala and Zwi, 2000). In November 1997 an international meeting on applied health research in complex emergencies was convened at the World Health Organization, and the Advisory Group on Research in Emergencies was established. Malaria was identified as one of the priority areas of communicable disease, and recommendations were specifically made to conduct research into the use of rapid diagnostic tests and prevention of transmission by use of insecticide-impregnated bed nets (World Health Organization, 1997b; Advisory Group on Research in Emergencies, 2000).[1]

Practical Considerations for Conducting Research

While the need for malaria-related research is evident, the feasibility of such projects should be considered prior to attempting to initiate research or special studies during a complex emergency. Outside researchers can be viewed as unwelcome burdens during emergencies, particularly during the initial phases of relief operations. However, if collaborative partnerships are forged from the beginning among those conducting the research, the nongovernmental organizations (NGOs) or other agencies providing the malaria control activities, and representatives of the intended beneficiary population, such studies will be feasible. Attention should be placed on the issues identified as problematic by field staff or the host government, and these should be relevant from a practical standpoint. Permission needs to be obtained from many levels—host governments, participating agencies,

---

[1]Reports from the advisory group's meetings and the research inventory can be accessed at <*http://www.who.int/eha*> or contact *eha@who.ch* for additional information.

the United Nations High Commissioner for Refugees or other lead relief organization, the participants themselves, and so forth. Consideration must be given to the practicalities of travel logistics, hiring of additional staff (both from the host government and from within the displaced population), the need for ongoing communication among all involved parties, cost effectiveness, and, particularly, security.

The research questions should be examined to determine whether they address only the displaced population or whether data gleaned from such studies have wider application to the host population (Williams and Bloland, 2001). For example, the authors of this monograph conducted antimalarial drug efficacy trials in refugee camps in western Tanzania in 1998. Those results complemented drug efficacy studies that had been conducted on the host population by the Ministry of Health. Together, those data helped to inform the decision to change the treatment of uncomplicated malaria in both the host country and the refugee population. However, a caveat was raised recently about competing tensions between the needs of the scientific community and those of the community involved. Ezard (2001a) provides an example of a refugee situation in which antimalarial drug efficacy data were urgently needed at the same time that local capacity needed to be strengthened to support self-determination. While attempting to recognize the needs for collaboration with the host country's health care professionals, prioritization of antimalarial drug efficacy studies did not match the local priority of establishing a new national health care system. Although ultimately successful in meeting both sets of priorities to some degree, Ezard stresses the need to recognize the underlying tensions between the achievement of short-term research goals and longer-term transfer of skills and development of local self-determination.

Roll Back Malaria has become very active in supporting and encouraging operational research related to malaria control and development and assessment of new tools and technologies appropriate for use in complex emergencies (see Allan and Guillet, 2002). Some of these technologies have been mentioned previously, such as wash-durable insecticide-treated nets and other insecticide-treatable emergency shelter materials. Many NGOs have recognized the need for additional malaria-specific operational research activities and are becoming very involved in conducting valuable research in emergency settings.

EXAMPLES OF PRIORITY AREAS FOR RESEARCH

Malaria Prevalence Surveys

If definitive diagnosis of malaria infection is not routine, rapid blood smear surveys of febrile patients can assist in evaluating the reliability of presumptive diagnoses. Surveys such as this are indicated in any area where malaria is believed to be transmitted and should be repeated during different times of the year, especially in areas where malaria transmission is believed to be seasonal. In Niger during the rainy season, for instance, over 99 percent of febrile patients were presumptively diagnosed as having malaria. But blood smears obtained from those patients confirmed malaria infection in only 62 percent. During the dry season, 79 percent of febrile patients were presumptively diagnosed as having malaria, but only 5.4 percent actually had parasites on blood smear (Olivar et al., 1991).

Rapid prevalence surveys can be done by simply obtaining and reading blood smears from 50 to 100 patients with fever or a history of fever who attend a health clinic. In areas where children are at greater risk than adults, as typically occurs in highly endemic areas, separate surveys based on age group should be done.

Therapy Efficacy Assessment

The best method to assess the efficacy of a chosen malaria therapy is by the in vivo test. The World Health Organization originally standardized the methodology, and there have since been numerous modifications. For the purposes of evaluating the efficacy of malaria therapy on a national level, emphasis has been on long follow-ups of patients (14 to 28 days or even longer). For the purposes of rapid assessment of therapy efficacy in an emergency setting, much useful information can be obtained by monitoring patients for even a minimal amount of time (such as 7 days), although longer follow-up of patients is preferable if at all possible. Suggested methods are presented in Appendix B.

Entomological Surveys

Any malaria control program that includes vector control or avoidance strategies requires a detailed entomological assessment to identify the primary vectors responsible for transmitting malaria. To ensure a valid assessment, these surveys must be conducted by a trained entomologist knowledgeable in malaria vectors and vector behavior.

Behavioral Research

As discussed in Chapter 8, little research has been done to answer behavioral questions related to malaria control activities in complex emergencies. In addition to the rapid assessments described earlier, other methods could be used, such as heath care facility surveys, with exit interviews to determine patients' understanding of their prescribed antimalarial medications or random surveys of households in displaced areas to inventory the types of drugs used for home or self-treatment of malaria.

Other research areas for which there are almost no data from displaced populations include patterns of treatment-seeking behaviors in a refugee camp or settlement area, the effect of economic dependency on the retention of distributed personal protective items (such as bed nets), patterns of compliance with antimalarial treatment during pregnancy, and understanding and correct usage of antimalarial drug treatment policies by relief health care workers. Samples of questions to guide sociobehavioral research can be found in the previous chapter. As noted previously, few NGOs have the internal capacity to conduct this type of research; such research should be guided by a trained social scientist.

Malaria in Pregnancy

Reproductive health and gender-related research have been identified as areas of pressing concern in emergency situations (World Health Organization, 1997b; Enarson, 1998; Palmer and Zwi, 1998; Palmer et al., 1999; Khaw et al., 2000). Studies of health care delivery could focus on better ways to integrate malaria prevention and treatment during pregnancy with other reproductive health-related interests, such as general management of complications related to pregnancy, the care of pregnant women infected with the human immunodeficiency virus, and the need to strengthen the linkages between traditional midwife care and antenatal services.

Questions pertaining to the feasibility and cost effectiveness of implementing preventive intermittent treatment for pregnant women also need to be addressed. A protocol to determine the rates of malaria parasitemia and anemia in women attending antenatal clinics and placental parasitemia and low-birthweight babies among women delivering in health care facilities is currently under development by the World Health Organization and the Centers for Disease Control and Prevention (M. Parise, Centers for Disease Control and Prevention, unpublished document, 2002). This protocol includes a rapid assessment guide to gather behavioral data related to sociobehavioral components of malaria and pregnancy. Although the protocol has been used only in nonemergency situations, it could be adapted for use in the more stable postemergency phase of displacement.

RECOMMENDATIONS

• Malaria prevalence surveys, therapy efficacy assessments, entomological surveys, and behavioral research should be considered essential routine activities to inform programmatic decisions.

• Findings of operational research should be documented in order to improve evidence-based humanitarian relief practice.

Operational Research: Key Points

• Operational research is necessary to make sound programmatic decisions.

• Priority areas for special studies include malaria prevalence surveys, therapy efficacy assessments, entomological surveys, and behavioral research.

• Developing collaborative partnerships among researchers, relief agency workers, and representatives of the affected communities is the best approach to obtaining this type of needed information.

10

Prophylaxis and Personal Protection for Relief Workers

Nonimmune personnel participating in humanitarian relief efforts need to protect themselves from malaria. The two principal strategies for doing so involve chemoprophylaxis and the use of personal protection measures. The choice of prophylaxis should be based on current knowledge of drug resistance patterns for the specific area. Because chloroquine resistance is widespread, chloroquine prophylaxis is useful only in Central America, Haiti, the Dominican Republic, and limited areas of the Middle East. One study of American Peace Corps volunteers exposed to chloroquine-resistant malaria demonstrated that prophylactic efficacy could be increased by combining chloroquine with proguanil, but the efficacy of this combination was still much below that obtainable with weekly mefloquine (Lobel et al., 1993). Among European travelers to East Africa, the prophylactic efficacy of chloroquine was 10 to 42 percent; for chloroquine combined with proguanil, 72 percent; and for weekly mefloquine, 91 percent (Steffen et al., 1993).

Use of amodiaquine and sulfadoxine/pyrimethamine for prophylaxis is not recommended due to a high incidence of serious, potentially fatal, adverse reactions. Currently, the only option for long-term chemoprophylaxis of nonimmune relief workers in most malarious areas of the world is mefloquine (in areas where mefloquine resistance is rare or does not exist). For shorter-term prophylaxis, doxycycline, or atovaquone/proguanil (Malarone) could be considered (see Table 10-1).

TABLE 10-1 Antimalarial Prophylaxis Regimens

Drug Name	Adult Dose	Estimated Cost[a] per Tablet
Mefloquine	228-250 mg (base)[c] once per week, starting 2 weeks before and during and 4 wks after exposure	$7.66
Malarone	1 tablet (250 mg atovaquone) per day, starting 2 days before and during and for 7 days after exposure	$3.95
Doxycycline	100 mg (salt) daily, starting 2 days before and during and 4 weeks after exposure	$0.39
Chloroquine	300 mg (base) once per week, starting 1 week before and during and 4 weeks after exposure	$4.50
Chloroquine + proguanil	Chloroquine as above plus proguanil 200 mg (salt) daily, continuing for 4 weeks after exposure	$4.50 (chloroquine) $0.03 (proguanil)

[a] Costs reflect average wholesale prices derived from the *Drug Topics Redbook* (Medical Economics Co., 1999) and the *International Drug Price Indicator Guide* (McFayden, 1999). Less expensive sources of some drugs exist internationally. These prices are intended for general comparative purposes only.
[b] Estimated cost includes pre- and postexposure doses (see text for explanation).

Personal protection measures are aimed at reducing human-mosquito contact during the evening and night. Personal protection measures include the use of insecticide-impregnated bed nets, insect repellents (especially those containing at least 30 percent DEET), protective clothing, and avoidance. Because no chemoprophylactic regimen is completely effective, a combination of preventive strategies is best. Up-to-date information regarding recommended chemoprophylaxis regimens and other prevention measures can be found on the following websites: Centers for Disease Control and Prevention recommendations (*<http://www.cdc.gov/travel/>*), World Health Organization recommendations (*<http://www.who.int/ith/>*); and Canadian recommendations (*<http://www.hc-sc.gc.ca/hpb/lcdc/publicat/ccdr/00vol26/26s2/index.html>*).

Estimated Cost[b] for 6 Months' Exposure	Comments/Cautions
$230 (30 tablets)	
$700 (177 tablets)	
$77 (198 tablets)	Not for use by pregnant women. Typically only used for limited duration of exposure.
$130 (29 tablets)	Only for use in Central America, northwest of Panama Canal, and island of Hispaniola. Price is for name-brand chloroquine; generics far less expensive.
$142 (29 tablets chloroquine + 396 tablets proguanil)	Addition of proguanil only marginally improves prophylactic efficacy of chloroquine, therefore not an advisable regimen for most instances. Proguanil not available in the U.S.

[c] Mefloquine marketed in the United States contains 228-mg base per tablet; mefloquine marketed in Europe contains a 250-mg base per tablet.

RECOMMENDATIONS

• Obtain current information on local drug resistance patterns when determining the most appropriate prophylaxis drug to recommend for relief workers.

• Either provide or facilitate provision of effective prophylactic medicines for relief workers.

• Train relief workers in the use of additional personal protection measures. Provide or facilitate the provision of materials needed for personal protection (such as insecticide-treated nets).

Chemoprophylaxis: Key Point

- Chemoprophylaxis and use of personal protective measures are necessary for protection of nonimmune relief personnel from malaria.

11

Return, Repatriation, or Resettlement of Displaced Populations

Many currently nonmalarious areas have mosquito species that are competent malaria vectors, and the introduction of a large population of gametocytemic individuals can cause the introduction or reintroduction of malaria (Slutsker et al., 1995; Bawden et al., 1995). Major population movements can dramatically alter the local epidemiology of malaria in endemic areas (Kazmi and Pandit, 2001). Additionally, population movement has also been identified as a major cause for the spread of drug-resistant malaria into new geographical areas (Teklehaimanot, 1986; Dar et al., 1993). Returning or relocated populations can place a large burden on the health care infrastructure of the receiving location and, if the receiving location is not malarious, existing provisions for dealing with large numbers of malaria patients may be inadequate (Paxton et al., 1996).

Therefore, plans for the resettlement or repatriation of displaced populations should be evaluated for the potential for introduction or reintroduction of malaria or multidrug-resistant malaria into the receiving area, and strategies to limit the movement of parasites along with relocating human populations should be considered. Options include the following:

- *Mass screening and selective treatment:* All relocating individuals should be screened with an appropriate diagnostic test (typically thick blood films), and those who are positive should be treated with an effective anti-malarial drug (including antirelapse or gametocytocidal agents, if indicated). However, individuals with subpatent infections or those with

P. vivax or *P. ovale* hypnozoites would not be identified and could become ill or act as a source of spread after relocation. Therefore, the capacity to diagnose and treat later would need to remain in place. This approach was recently used successfully for approximately 900 Vietnamese Montangard refugees being relocated from camps in Cambodia to the United States (Centers for Disease Control and Prevention, unpublished data). Because of an expected low prevalence of malaria in this population and limited treatment options due to drug resistance patterns in the region, all refugees were screened during routine pre-departure health screening with rapid diagnostic tests (with thick blood smears obtained as back-up). Only those proven to be positive were treated with a combination of mefloquine and artesunate. Because exposure to *P. vivax* was expected to be common, however, the entire population was treated presumptively with 14 days of primaquine (after being screened for G6PD deficiency) after arrival in the United States.

• *Mass presumptive treatment:* Everyone in a population should be treated presumptively with an effective antimalarial (including antirelapse agents if indicated). This option may be appropriate if the prevalence of malaria infection in the relocating population is high (Paxton et al., 1996; Centers for Disease Control and Prevention, 1998). Treatment should be done as close to the time of departure as possible to avoid the chance of reinfection before transit.

• *Fever surveillance and case management:* Surveillance (active or passive, as required) should be set up in the receiving area to identify individuals with febrile illness. These individuals should be diagnosed and treated with an effective antimalarial as needed. This option may be most appropriate among populations where initial malaria prevalence is very low, postrelocation surveillance is possible, and facilities capable of diagnosing and treating malaria are readily accessible. This might also be the least attractive option for populations with a high level of acquired malaria immunity. (Relatively few infections would be associated with fever and would therefore not be picked up by fever surveillance.)

Decisions regarding which option is the most cost effective must take into account a number of factors, including the prevalence of malaria in the displaced population; the level of asymptomatic infection; the risk of introduced malaria in the receiving area; the cost, efficacy, safety, and ease of use of the chosen malaria treatment; and the cost of diagnosing and treating malaria in the receiving area. These variables differ greatly from situation

Impact of Resettlement and Repatriation on Malaria Resurgence: Key Points

- Resettlement or repatriation of displaced populations can potentially introduce or reintroduce malaria or multidrug-resistant malaria into the receiving area.
- Clinical malaria can be a problem among resettled populations long after relocation.
- Strategies for limiting the movement of malaria parasites along with relocating humans and minimizing postrelocation morbidity and mortality include mass screening and selective treatment, mass presumptive treatment, and fever surveillance and case management.

to situation. For example, partly because of the very high cost of malaria treatment in the United States, the prevalence threshold for making mass treatment prior to relocation a more cost-effective approach for refugees being relocated from East Africa to the United States was as low as 2 percent (Cookson, 1999).

Another situation requiring planning is when displaced populations return to an endemic area after residing in a nonendemic area of refuge. Even after a relatively short period of time unexposed, acquired immunity can be diminished and, as a result, returnees can be at increased risk of severe illness and death. Adequate preparations should be made prior to arrival to educate returnees about the risks, to offer guidance and advice about the use of personal protection measures, to distribute insecticide-impregnated bed nets (if appropriate), and to provide effective antimalarial treatment to anyone exhibiting an illness suggestive of malaria.

RECOMMENDATION

- Consider interventions to address malaria, including curative and preventive services, at the point of departure or arrival. Responsibility for the provision of effective malaria control does not end with repatriation or resettlement.

Recommendations for Improving
Malaria Control Services

• Malaria control services can be improved by instituting a task force representing all involved agencies with the goal of improving the integration and coordination of malaria control strategies.

• Improving public health malaria practices should involve representatives from the displaced community, the host community, and the humanitarian relief community.

12

Improving Malaria Control in Complex Emergencies

PRACTICAL CONSIDERATIONS FOR IMPLEMENTING MALARIA CONTROL

Implementing malaria control in a complex emergency generally requires concerted attention to coordination, communication, and organization because of the number of agencies involved, the fluidity with which emergency situations change, the limited consensus often seen among agencies regarding a plan of action for malaria control, and the lack of a single clearly identified organizing agency or committee to lead the effort. Criticism has frequently been leveled at nongovernmental organizations (NGOs) and the United Nations Office of the High Commissioner for Refugees (UNHCR) over poor programmatic planning, limited assessments, lack of coordination among and within relief agencies, and marginal management skills (Walkup, 1997; Seaman, 1999; Zetter, 1999). The need for a malaria control program plan that is well integrated and accepted by all participating agencies is particularly important in situations of delicate political sensitivities, such as when the malaria policy for a displaced population differs from the standard national policy.

One approach to strengthening malaria control program planning is to establish, at the beginning stages of an emergency, a joint working group whose mandate is to coordinate all primary health care services. From this larger group, a task force or committee could be formed to concentrate on how to best prevent and manage malaria. These groups should consist of representatives from any agency involved in control activities (case management, vector control, health education, water, and sanitation), along with camp officials, the UNHCR and other United Nations agencies, NGOs, the host government (especially the National Malaria Control Program, if one is in existence), the local host community, and the displaced community. This group should be convened on a regular basis, and all partners should be represented from the beginning. Each agency's role and stake in malaria control should be clear to the other partners.

ADAPTATION OF THE PUBLIC NUTRITION APPROACH TO MALARIA CONTROL

Given the role that context and sociocultural behaviors play in malaria control, it is time to rethink additional ways to improve malaria control in complex emergencies. Adapting the "Public Nutrition" approach in malaria control might be an option. Using multidisciplinary approaches, registered public health nutritionists use theories of nutrition and social science to critically examine the social, political, and economic determinants of malnutrition (Borrel and Salama, 1999; Landman, 1999; Young, 1999). This approach would move the dialogue beyond standard ways of using malaria-related morbidity and mortality numbers to describe those affected by asking and attempting to answer the question: "Why are they affected?" Rather than examining only the willingness of people to engage in malaria control, this approach would also look at their ability to alter behaviors related to malaria, given the political, social, and economic constraints they face. Adapting the principles of public nutrition and expanding our understanding of the macro-level forces that affect the ability to implement quality malaria control programs will strengthen public health practices.

COMMUNITY INVOLVEMENT IN MALARIA CONTROL

Although use of the terms "community involvement" and "community mobilization" has become ubiquitous in public health discourses, stressing the need to have a displaced community fully represented is warranted. In the context of a complex emergency, "community" should be broadened to include four groups: members of the displaced community, members of the host community, representatives from the humanitarian relief community, and representatives of the government of the country of asylum. Each of these separate communities may have differing perspectives, interests, needs, and priorities with regard to malaria control. It is essential that malaria control activities be developed collaboratively and that an integrated plan of action reflects the concerns and resources of all members of the involved parties. Attention to the cultural milieu of the situation, good communication, and creative approaches to integrating community participation will enhance malaria control programs.

As mentioned earlier, representation on the joint malaria control working committee and use of rapid assessment techniques are two ways to involve communities. Other areas include incorporating traditional healers into clinical rounds; developing economic incentive programs, particularly for preventive measures; using community health care workers to assist with vulnerable populations; training local health care workers to interpret data they routinely collect as a first step in designing community-based control measures; and linking malaria control activities to other community-based activities that are in process and accepted.

RECOMMENDATIONS

- Form a task force for integrated malaria control as early in an emergency as possible.
- Include representatives from all involved communities (host country, displaced population, and relief organizations) on the task force.
- Use multidisciplinary approaches to develop better malaria control strategies.

References

Abisudjak, B., and R. Kotanegara
　1989　Transmigration and vector-borne diseases in Indonesia. Pp. 207-223 in *Demography and Vector-borne Diseases*, M.W. Service, ed. Boca Raton, FL: CRC Press.

Advisory Group on Research in Emergencies
　2000　*Advisory Group on Research in Emergencies Brief 12-8-00*. Geneva: World Health Organization.

Alemayehu, T., Y. Ye-ebiyo, T.A. Ghebreyesus, K.H. Witten, A. Bosman, and A. Teklehaimonot
　1998　Malaria, schistosomiasis, and intestinal helminths in relation to microdams in Tigray, northern Ethiopia. *Parassitologia* 40:259-267.

Allan, R., and P. Guillet
　2002　Roll Back Malaria: Challenges in Complex Emergencies. Available: *<http://mosquito.who.int/cmc_upload/0/000/015/262/iatr_jan2002_1.htm>* [November 5, 2002].

Alonso, P.L., S.W. Lindsay, J. Armstrong Schellenberg, K. Keita, P. Gomez, F.C. Shenton, A.G. Hill, P.H. David, G. Fegan, K. Cham, and B.M. Greenwood
　1993　A malaria control trial using insecticide-treated bed nets and targeted chemo-prophylaxis in a rural area of the Gambia, West Africa. 6. The impact of the interventions on mortality and morbidity from malaria. *Transactions of the Royal Society of Tropical Medicine and Hygiene* 87(Suppl. 2):37-44.

Anonymous
　1999　El Niño and associated outbreaks of severe malaria in highland populations in Irian Jaya, Indonesia: A review and epidemiologic perspective. *Southeast Asian Journal of Tropical Medicine and Public Health* 30:608-619.

Baird, J.K., D.J. Fryauff, H. Basri, M.J. Bangs, B. Subianto, I. Wiady, Purnomo, B. Leksana, S. Masbar, T.L. Richie, T.R. Jones, E. Tjitra, F.S. Wignall, and S.L. Hoffman
  1995 Primaquine for prophylaxis against malaria among nonimmune transmigrants in Irian Jaya, Indonesia. *American Journal of Tropical Medicine and Hygiene* 52(6):479-484.
Banatvala, N., and A. Zwi
  2000 Public health and humanitarian interventions: Developing the evidence base. *British Medical Journal* 321:101-105.
Barat, L., J. Chippa, M. Kolczak, and T. Sukwa
  1999 Does the availability of blood slide microscopy for malaria at health centers improve the management of persons with fever in Zambia? *American Journal of Tropical Medicine and Hygiene* 60:1024-1030.
Bawden, M.P., D.D. Slaten, and J.D. Malone
  1995 *Falciparum* malaria in a displaced Haitian population. *Transactions of the Royal Society of Tropical Medicine and Hygiene* 89:600-603.
Bayley, A.M., and I.G. Macreadie
  2002 Folic acid antagonism of sulfa drug treatments. *Trends in Parasitology* 18:49-50.
Beebe, J.
  1995 Basic concepts and techniques of rapid appraisal. *Human Organization* 53:42-51.
Bermejo, A., and H. Veeken
  1992 Insecticide-impregnated bed nets for malaria control: A review of the field trials. *Bulletin of the World Health Organization* 70:293-296.
Björkman, A., and P.A. Phillips-Howard
  1990 The epidemiology of drug-resistant malaria. *Transactions of the Royal Society of Tropical Medicine and Hygiene* 84:177-180.
Bloland, P.B., and M. Ettling
  1999 Making malaria-treatment policy in the face of drug resistance. *Annals of Tropical Medicine and Parasitology* 93:5-23.
Bloland, P.B., E.M. Lackritz, P.N. Kazembe, J.B. Were, R. Steketee, and C.C. Campbell
  1993 Beyond chloroquine: Implications of drug resistance for evaluating malaria therapy efficacy and treatment policy in Africa. *Journal of Infectious Diseases* 167:932-937.
Bloland, P.B., M. Ettling, and S. Meek
  2000 Combination therapy for malaria in Africa: Hype or hope? *Bulletin of the World Health Organization* 78:1378-1388.
Bojang, K.A., S. Obaro, L.A. Morison, and B.M. Greenwood
  2000 A prospective evaluation of a clinical algorithm for the diagnosis of malaria in Gambian children. *Tropical Medicine and International Health* 5:231-236.
Borrel, A., and P. Salama
  1999 Public nutrition from an approach to a discipline: Concern's nutrition case studies in complex emergencies. *Disasters* 23:326-342.
Bouma, M.J., and H.J. van der Kaay
  1994 Epidemic malaria in India and the El Niño Southern Oscillation. *Lancet* 344:1638-1639.

Bouma, M., and M. Rowland
    1995   Failure of passive zooprophylaxis: Cattle ownership in Pakistan is associated with a higher prevalence of malaria. *Transactions of the Royal Society of Tropical Medicine and Hygiene* 89:351-353.
Bouma, M.J., G. Poveda, W. Rojas, D. Chavasse, M. Quiñones, J. Cox, and J. Patz
    1997   Predicting high-risk years for malaria in Colombia using parameters of El Niño Southern Oscillation. *Tropical Medicine and International Health* 2:1122-1127.
Brinkmann, U., and A. Brinkmann
    1995   Economic aspects of the use of impregnated nets for malaria control. *Bulletin of the World Health Organization* 73:651-658.
Brockman, A., R.N. Price, M. van Vugt, D.G. Heppner, D. Walsh, P. Sookto, T. Wimonwattrawatee, S. Looareesuwan, N.J. White, and F. Nosten
    2000   *Plasmodium falciparum* antimalarial drug susceptibility on the north-western border of Thailand during five years of extensive use of artesunate-mefloquine. *Transactions of the Royal Society of Tropical Medicine and Hygiene* 94:537-544.
Bruce-Chwatt, L.J.
    1985   *Essential Malariology*, 2nd ed. New York: John Wiley & Sons.
Brundtland, G.H.
    2000   Editorial: Mental health of refugees, internally displaced persons and other populations affected by conflict. *Acta Psychiatrica Scandinavica* 102:159-161.
Bunnag, D., and T. Harinasuta
    1987   Quinine and quinidine in malaria in Thailand. *Acta Leidensia* 55:163-166.
Bureau for Refugee Programs
    1985   *Assessment Manual for Refugee Emergencies.* Washington, DC: U.S. Department of State.
Burkholder, B.T., and M.J. Toole
    1995   Evolution of complex disasters. *Lancet* 346:1012-1015.
Burkle, F.M.
    1999   Fortnightly review: Lessons learnt and future expectations of complex emergencies. *British Medical Journal* 319:422-426.
Campbell, C.C.
    1991   Challenges facing antimalarial therapy in Africa. *Journal of Infectious Diseases* 163:1207-1211.
Centers for Disease Control
    1992   Famine-affected, refugee, and displaced populations: Recommendations for public health issues. *Morbidity and Mortality Weekly Report* 41(RR-13, 14):1-76.
Centers for Disease Control and Prevention
    1996   Morbidity and mortality surveillance in Rwandan refugees—Burundi and Zaire, 1994. *Morbidity and Mortality Weekly Report* 45:104-107.
    1998   Enhanced medical assessment strategy for Barawan Somali refugees—Kenya, 1997. *Morbidity and Mortality Weekly Report* 46:1250-1254.
    2000   *Health Information for the International Traveler 2001-2002.* Atlanta: U.S. Department of Health and Human Services, Public Health Service.
    2001   Updated guidelines for evaluating public health surveillance systems. *Morbidity and Mortality Weekly Report* 50(32)(RR-14), 1-35.

Cham, M., B. Olaleye, U. D'Alessandro, M. Aikins, B. Cham, N. Maine, L. Williams, A. Mills, and B. Greenwood

1997   The impact of charging for insecticide on the Gambian national impregnated bednet programme. *Health Policy and Planning* 12:240-247.

Chambers, R.

1992   *Rural Appraisal: Rapid, Relaxed and Participatory.* Institute of Development Studies. Discussion Paper 311. Brighton, England: University of Sussex.

Chareonviriyaphap, T., M.J. Bangs, and S. Ratanathan

2000   Status of malaria in Thailand. *Southeast Asian Journal of Tropical Medicine and Public Health* 31:225-237.

Choi, H.W., J.G. Breman, S.M. Teutsch, S. Liu, A.W. Hightower, and J.D. Sexton

1995   The effectiveness of insecticide-impregnated bed nets in reducing cases of malaria infection: A meta-analysis of published results. *American Journal of Tropical Medicine and Hygiene* 52:377-382.

Collins, W.E., and G.M. Jeffery

1996   Primaquine resistance in *Plasmodium vivax. American Journal of Tropical Medicine and Hygiene* 55:243-249.

Cookson, S.

1999   Enhanced Refugee Health Assessment. Oral presentation, Medical Screening International Meeting, International Organization for Migration, Geneva, Switzerland, Oct. 8-9.

Corbett, E.L., R.W. Steketee, F.O. ter Kuile, A.S. Latif, A. Kamali, and R.J. Hayes

2002   HIV-1/AIDS and the control of other infectious diseases in Africa. *Lancet* 359(9324):2177-2187.

Cornwall, A., and R. Jewkes

1995   What is participatory research? *Social Science and Medicine* 41:1667-1676.

Craig, M.H., and B.L. Sharp

1997   Comparative evaluation of four techniques for the diagnosis of *Plasmodium falciparum* infections. *Transactions of the Royal Society of Tropical Medicine and Hygiene* 91:279-282.

Crawley, J.

2001   Reducing deaths from malaria among children: The pivotal role of prompt, effective treatment. *Africa Health* (Suppl. September 25).

Cromwell, G.

1988   Note on the role of expatriate administrators in agency-assisted refugee programs. *Journal of Refugee Studies* 1:297-307.

Curtis, C.F., and A.E.P. Mnzava

2000   Comparison of house spraying and insecticide-treated nets for malaria control. *Bulletin of the World Health Organization* 78:1389-1400.

Cuzin-Ouattara, N., A.H.A. van den Broek, A. Habluetzel, A. Diabaté, E. Sanogo-Ilboudo, D.A. Diallo, S.N. Cousens, and F. Esposito

1999   Wide-scale installation of insecticide-treated curtains confers high levels of protection against malaria transmission in a hyperendemic area of Burkina Faso. *Transactions of the Royal Society of Tropical Medicine and Hygiene* 93:473-479.

D'Alessandro, U., B. Olaleye, W. McGuire, P. Langerock, S. Bennett, M.K. Aikins, M.C. Thomson, M.K. Cham, B.A. Cham, and B.M. Greenwood
  1995   Mortality and morbidity from malaria in Gambian children after introduction of an impregnated bednet programme. *Lancet* 345:479-483.

Dar, F.K., R. Bayoumi, T. Al Karmi, A. Shalabi, F. Beidas, and M.M. Hussein
  1993   Status of imported malaria in a control zone of the United Arab Emirates bordering an area of unstable malaria. *Transactions of the Royal Society of Tropical Medicine and Hygiene* 87:617-619.

David, J., L. Zakus, and C.L. Lysack
  1998   Review article: Revisiting community participation. *Health Policy and Planning* 13:1-12.

Day, N.P.J., N.H. Phu, N.T.H. Mai, T.T.H. Chau, P.P. Loc, L. Van Chuong, D.X. Sinh, P. Holloway, T.T. Hien, and N.J. White
  2000   The pathophysiologic and prognostic significance of acidosis in severe adult malaria. *Critical Care Medicine* 28:1833-1840.

de Andrade, A.L.S.S., C.M.T. Martelli, R.M. Oliveira, J.R. Arias, F. Zicker, and L. Pang
  1995   High prevalence of asymptomatic malaria in gold mining areas in Brazil. *Clinical Infectious Diseases* 20:475.

Decludt, B., B. Pecoul, P. Biberson, R. Lang, and S. Imivithaya
  1991   Malaria surveillance among the displaced Karen population in Thailand April 1984 to February 1989, Mae Sot, Thailand. *Southeast Asian Journal of Tropical Medicine and Public Health* 22:504-508.

Defo, B.K.
  1995   Epidemiology and control of infant and early childhood malaria: A competing risks analysis. *International Journal of Epidemiology* 24:204-217.

Dick, B., and S. Simmonds
  1983   Refugee health care: Similar but different? *Disasters* 7:291-303.

Djimdé, A., O.K. Doumbo, R.W. Steketee, and C.V. Plowe
  2001   Application of a molecular marker for surveillance of chloroquine-resistant falciparum malaria. *Lancet* 358:890-891.

Doherty, J.F., A.D. Sadiq, L. Bayo, A. Alloueche, P. Olliaro, P. Milligan, L. von Seidlein, and M. Pinder
  1999   A randomized safety and efficacy trial of artesunate plus sulfadoxine-pyrimethamine vs. sulfadoxine-pyrimethamine alone for the treatment of uncomplicated malaria in Gambian children. *Transactions of the Royal Society of Tropical Medicine and Hygiene* 93(5):543-546.

Dolan, G., F.O. ter Kuile, V. Jacoutot, N.J. White, C. Luxemburger, L. Malankirii, T. Chongsuphajaisiddhi, and F. Nosten
  1993   Bed nets for the prevention of malaria and anaemia in pregnancy. *Transactions of the Royal Society of Tropical Medicine and Hygiene* 87(6):620-626.

Duffield, M.
  1994   The political economy of internal war: Asset transfer, complex emergencies and international aid. Pp. 50-69 in *War and Hunger: Rethinking International Responses to Complex Emergencies*, J. Macrae and A. Zwi, eds. London: Zed Books.

Enarson, E.
1998 Through women's eyes: A gendered research agenda for disaster social science. *Disasters* 22:157-173.

English, M., R. Sauerwein, C. Waruiru, M. Mosobo, J. Obeiro, B. Lowe, and K. Marsh
1997 Acidosis in severe childhood malaria. *Quarterly Journal of Medicine* 90:263-270.

Enwere, G.C., M.O. Ota, and S.K. Obaro
1999 The host response in malaria and depression of defense against tuberculosis. *Annals of Tropical Medicine and Parasitology* 93:669-678.

Ezard, N.
2001a Research in complex emergencies. *Lancet* 357:149.
2001b *Emergency Malaria Control for Refugee Affected Populations, Kissidougou, Dabola and Guéckedou, Guinea.* (Provisional Report) Roll Back Malaria Complex Emergencies, April 7-June 6, 2001. Geneva: World Health Organization.

Fortier, B., P. Delplace, J.F. Dubremetz, F. Ajana, and A. Vernes
1987 Enzyme immunoassay for detection of antigen in acute *Plasmodium falciparum* malaria. *European Journal of Clinical Microbiology* 6:596-598.

Foster, S.
1995 Treatment of malaria outside the formal health services. *Journal of Tropical Medicine and Hygiene* 98:29-34.

Gilles, H.M.
1993 Epidemiology of malaria. Pp. 124-163 in *Bruce-Chwatt's Essential Malariology, 3rd Edition,* H.M. Gilles and D.A. Warrell, eds. New York: Oxford University Press.

Githeko, A.K., S.W. Lindsay, U.E. Confalonieri, and J.A. Patz
2000 Climate change and vector-borne diseases: A regional analysis. *Bulletin of the World Health Organization* 78:1136-1147.

Glass, R.I., W. Cates, P. Nieburg, C. Davis, R. Russbach, H. Nothdurft, S. Peel, and R. Turnbull
1980 Rapid assessment of health status and preventive-medicine needs of newly arrived Kampuchean refugees, Sa Kaeo, Thailand. *Lancet* (8173):868-872.

Goma Epidemiology Group
1995 Public health impact of Rwandan refugee crisis: What happened in Goma, Zaire, in July 1994? *Lancet* 345:339-344.

Goodhand, J., and D. Hulme
1999 From wars to complex political emergencies: Understanding conflict and peace-building in the new world disorder. *Third World Quarterly* 20(1):13-26.

Goodman, C.A., P.G. Coleman, and A.J. Mills
1999 Cost-effectiveness of malaria control in sub-Saharan Africa. *Lancet* 354:378-385.

Goodman, C.A., A.E.P. Mnzava, S.S. Dlamini, B.L. Sharp, D.J. Mthembu, and J.K. Gumede
2001 Comparison of the cost and cost-effectiveness of insecticide-treated bednets and residual house-spraying in Kwa-Zulu Natal, South Africa. *Tropical Medicine and International Health* 6:280-295.

Greenberg, A.E., M. Ntumbanzondo, N. Ntula, L. Mawa, J. Howell, and F. Davachi
1989 Hospital-based surveillance of malaria-related paediatric morbidity and mortality in Kinshasa, Zaire. *Bulletin of the World Health Organization* 67:189-196.

Greenwood, A.M., B.M. Greenwood, A.K. Bradley, and P.A.S. Ball
1981 Enhancement of the immune response to meningococcal polysaccharides vaccine

in a malaria endemic area by administration of chloroquine. *Annals of Tropical Medicine and Parasitology* 75:261-263.

Greenwood, B.M.
  1987   Asymptomatic malaria infections. Do they matter? *Parasitology Today* 3:206-214.

Greenwood, B.M., A.K. Bradley, A.M. Greenwood, P. Byass, K. Jammeh, K. Marsh, S. Tulloch, F.S. Oldfield, and R. Hayes
  1987   Mortality and morbidity from malaria among children in a rural area of the Gambia, West Africa. *Transactions of the Royal Society of Tropical Medicine and Hygiene* 81(3):478-486.

Greenwood, B., and T. Mutabingwa
  2002   Malaria in 2002. *Nature* 415(6872):670-672.

Guiguemde, T.R., F. Dao, V. Curtis, A. Traore, B. Dondo, J. Testa, and J.B. Ouedraogo
  1994   Household expenditures on malaria prevention and treatment for families in the town of Bobo-Dioulasso, Burkina Faso. *Transactions of the Royal Society of Tropical Medicine and Hygiene* 88:285-287.

Guillet, P., D. Alnwick, M.K. Cham, M. Neira, M. Zaim, D. Heymann, and K. Mukelabai
  2001   Long-lasting treated mosquito nets: A breakthrough in malaria prevention. *Bulletin of the World Health Organization* 79(10):998.

Habluetzel, A., D.A. Diallo, F. Esposito, L. Lamizana, F. Pagnoni, C. Lengeler, C. Traore, and S.N. Cousens
  1997   Do insecticide-impregnated curtains reduce all-cause child mortality in Burkina Faso? *Tropical Medicine and International Health* 2:855-862.

Habluetzel, A., N. Cuzin, D.A. Diallo, I. Nebié, S. Belem, S. Cousens, and F. Esposito
  1999   Insecticide-treated curtains reduce the prevalence and intensity of malaria infection in Burkina Faso. *Tropical Medicine and International Health* 4:557-564.

Hawley, W.A., P.A. Phillips-Howard, F.O. ter Kuile, D.J. Terlouw, J.M. Vulule, M. Ombok, B.L. Nahlen, J.E. Gimnig, S.K. Kariuki, M.S. Kolczak, and A.W. Hightower
  In   Community-wide effects of permethrin-treated bednets on child mortality and
  press malaria morbidity in western Kenya. *American Journal Tropical Medicine and Hygiene.*

Hendrikse, R.G., A.H. Hasan, L.O. Olumide, and A. Akinkunmi
  1971   Malaria in early childhood. *Annals of Tropical Medicine and Parasitology* 65:1-20.

Hewitt, S., M. Kamal, N. Muhammad, and M. Rowland
  1994   An entomological investigation of the likely impact of cattle ownership on malaria in an Afghan refugee camp in the north west frontier province of Pakistan. *Medical and Veterinary Entomology* 8:160-164.

Hewitt, S., M. Rowland, N. Muhammad, M. Kamal, and E. Kemp
  1995   Pyrethroid-sprayed tents for malaria control: An entomologic evaluation in Pakistan. *Medical and Veterinary Entomology* 9:344-352.

Hoffman, I.F., C.S. Jere, T.E. Taylor, P. Munthali, J.R. Dyer, J.J. Wirima, S.J. Rogerson, N. Kumwenda, J.J. Eron, S.A. Fiscus, H. Chakraborty, T.E. Taha, M.S. Cohen, and M.E. Molyneux
  1999   The effect of *Plasmodium falciparum* malaria on HIV-1 RNA blood plasma concentration. *AIDS* 13(4):487-494.

Howard, S.C., J. Omumbo, C. Nevill, E.S. Some, C.A. Donnelly, and R.W. Snow
  2000   Evidence for a mass community effect of insecticide-treated bednets on the

incidence of malaria on the Kenyan coast. *Transactions of the Royal Society of Tropical Medicine and Hygiene* 94(4):357-360.

Jaspers, S., and J. Shoham

1999 Targeting the vulnerable: A review of the necessity and feasibility of targeting vulnerable households. *Disasters* 23:359-372.

Jonkman, A., R.A. Chibwe, C.O. Khoromana, U.L. Liabunya, M.E. Chaponda, G.E. Kandiero, M.E. Molyneux, and T.E. Taylor

1995 Cost-saving through microscopy-based versus presumptive diagnosis of malaria in adult outpatients in Malawi. *Bulletin of the World Health Organization* 73(2):223-227.

Kachur, S.P., S. Abdulla, K. Barnes, H. Mshinda, D. Durrheim, A. Kitua, and P. Bloland

2001 Letter to the editors. *Tropical Medicine and International Health* 6:324-325.

Kamol-Ratanakul, P., and C. Prasittisuk

1992 The effectiveness of permethrin-impregnated bed nets against malaria for migrant workers in eastern Thailand. *American Journal of Tropical Medicine and Hygiene* 47:305-309.

Kaneko, A., G. Taleo, M. Kalkoa, S. Yamar, T. Kobayakawa, and A. Björkman

2000 Malaria eradication on islands. *Lancet* 356:1560-1564.

Karch, S., N. Asidi, Z.M. Manzambi, and J.J. Salaun

1992 Efficacy of *Bacillus sphaericus* against the malaria vector *Anopheles gambiae* and other mosquitoes in swamps and rice fields in Zaire. *Journal of the American Mosquito Control Association* 8:376-380.

Kassankogno, Y., R. Allan, and C. Delcollette

2000 *Management of Malaria in Epidemic Affected Areas of Burundi.* Geneva: World Health Organization/Roll Back Malaria Complex Emergency Network/Roll Back Malaria Epidemic Prevention and Control Network.

Kazmi, J.H., and K. Pandit

2001 Disease and dislocation: The impact of refugee movements on the geography of malaria in NWFP, Pakistan. *Social Science and Medicine* 52:1043-1055.

Kere, J.F., and N.K. Kere

1992 Bed-nets or spraying? Cost analyses of malaria control in the Solomon Islands. *Health Policy and Planning* 7:382-386.

Khaw, A., P. Salama, B. Burkholder, and T.J. Dondero

2000 HIV risk and prevention in emergency-affected populations: A review. *Disasters* 24:181-197.

Khusmith, S., S. Tharavanij, R. Kasemsuth, C. Vejvongvarn, and D. Bunnag

1987 Two-site immunoradiometric assay for detection of *Plasmodium falciparum* antigen in blood using monoclonal and polyclonal antibodies. *Journal of Clinical Microbiology* 25:1467-1471.

Kinde-Gazard, O.J., I.I. Gnahoui, and A. Massougbodji

2000 The risk of malaria transmission by blood transfusion at Cotonou, Benin. *Sante* 10:389-392.

Kloos, H.

1990 Health aspects of resettlement in Ethiopia. *Social Science and Medicine* 30:643-656.

Knudsen, A.B., and R. Slooff

1992   Vector-borne disease problems in rapid urbanization: New approaches to vector control. *Bulletin of the World Health Organization* 70:1-6.

Koram, K.A., S. Bennett, J.H. Adiamah, and B.M. Greenwood

1995a   Socio-economic risk factors for malaria in a peri-urban area of the Gambia. *Transactions of the Royal Society of Tropical Medicine and Hygiene* 89:146-150.

1995b   Socio-economic determinants are not major risk factors for severe malaria in Gambian children. *Transactions of the Royal Society of Tropical Medicine and Hygiene* 89:151-154.

Krishna, S., T. Planche, T. Agbenyega, C. Woodrow, D. Agranoff, G. Bedu-Addo, A.K. Owusu-Ofori, J.A. Appiah, S. Ramanathan, S.M. Mansor, and V. Navaratnam

2001   Bioavailability and preliminary clinical efficacy of intrarectal artesunate in Ghanaian children with moderate malaria. *Antimicrobial Agents and Chemotherapy* 45:509-516.

Kroeger, A., A. Gerhardus, G. Kruger, M. Mancheno, and K. Pesse

1997   The contribution of repellent soap to malaria control. *American Journal of Tropical Medicine and Hygiene* 56:580-584.

Kwiatkowski, D.

1990   Tumour necrosis factor, fever and fatality in falciparum malaria. *Immunology Letters* 25:213-216.

Lackritz, E.M.

1998   Prevention of HIV transmission by blood transfusion in the developing world: Achievements and continuing challenges. *AIDS* 12(Suppl. A):S81-S86.

Lackritz, E.M., C.C. Campbell, T.K. Ruebush II, A.W. Hightower, W. Wakube, R.W. Steketee, and J.B. Were

1992   Effect of blood transfusion on survival among children in a Kenyan hospital. *Lancet* 340(8818):524-528.

Lackritz, E.M., A.W. Hightower, J.R. Zucker, T.K. Ruebush, C.O. Onudi, R.W. Steketee, J.B.O. Were, E. Patrick, and C.C. Campbell

1997   Longitudinal evaluation of severely anemic children in Kenya: The effect of transfusion on mortality and hematologic recovery. *AIDS* 11:1487-1494.

Landman, J.

1999   Food aid in emergencies: A case for wheat? *Proceedings of the Nutrition Society* 58:355-361.

Lell, B., J-F. Faucher, M.A. Missinou, S. Bormann, O. Dangelmaier, J. Horton, and P.G. Kremsner

2000   Malaria chemoprophylaxis with tafenoquine: A randomized study. *Lancet* 355:2041-2045.

Lengeler, C.

1998   Insecticide treated bednets and curtains for malaria control (Cochrane Review). Abstract from *The Cochrane Library* Issue 4. Oxford: Update Software Ltd. Available: <*http://www.update-software.com/abstracts/ab000363.htm*> [September 25, 2002].

Levine, R.A., S.C. Wardlaw, and C.L. Patton

1989   Detection of haematoparasites using quantitative buffy coat analysis tubes. *Parasitology Today* 5:132-133.

Lindblade, K.A., E.D. Walker, A.W. Onapa, J. Katungu, and M.L. Wilson
  1999 Highland malaria in Uganda: Prospective analysis of an epidemic associated with El Niño. *Transactions of the Royal Society of Tropical Medicine and Hygiene* 93:480-487.
Lindsay, S.W., J.H. Adiamah, J.E. Miller, and J.R.M. Armstrong
  1991 Pyrethroid-treated bed net effects on mosquitoes of the *Anopheles gambiae* complex in the Gambia. *Medical and Veterinary Entomology* 5:477-483.
Lindsay, S.W., R. Bodker, R. Malima, H.A. Msangeni, and W. Kisinza
  2000 Effect of 1997-98 El Niño on highland malaria in Tanzania. *Lancet* 355:989-990.
Lobel, H.O., M. Miani, T. Eng, K.W. Bernard, A.W. Hightower, and C.C. Campbell
  1993 Long-term malaria prophylaxis with weekly mefloquine. *Lancet* 341:848-851.
Looareesuwan, S., C. Viravan, H.K. Webster, D.E. Kyle, D.B. Hutchinson, and C.J. Canfield
  1996a Clinical studies of atovaquone, alone or in combination with other antimalarial drugs for the treatment of acute uncomplicated malaria in Thailand. *American Journal of Tropical Medicine and Hygiene* 54(1):62-66.
Looareesuwan, S., P. Olliaro, D. Kyle, and W. Wernsdorfer
  1996b Pyronaridine. *Lancet* 347:1189-1190.
Luby, S.P., P.N. Kazembe, S.C. Redd, C. Ziba, O.C. Nwanyanwu, A.W. Hightower, C. Franco, L. Chitsulo, J.J. Wirima, and M.A. Olivar
  1995 Using clinical signs to diagnose anaemia in African children. *Bulletin of the World Health Organization* 73:477-482.
Luxemburger, C., W.A. Perea, G. Delmas, C. Pruja, B. Pecoul, and A. Moren
  1994 Permethrin-impregnated bed nets for the prevention of malaria in schoolchildren on the Thai-Burmese border. *Transactions of the Royal Society of Tropical Medicine and Hygiene* 88:155-159.
Luxemburger, C., M. van Vugt, S. Jonathan, R. McGready, S. Looareesuwan, N.J. White, and F. Nosten
  1999 Treatment of vivax malaria on the western border of Thailand. *Transactions of the Royal Society of Tropical Medicine and Hygiene* 93:433-438.
Mabey, D.C., A. Brown, and B.M. Greenwood
  1987 *Plasmodium falciparum* malaria and *Salmonella* infections in Gambian children. *Journal of Infectious Diseases* 155:1319-1321.
Mabeza, G.F., G. Biemba, A.G. Brennan, V.M. Moyo, P.E. Thuma, and V.R. Gordeuk
  1998 The association of pallor with haemoglobin concentration and mortality in severe malaria. *Annals of Tropical Medicine and Parasitology* 92:663-669.
MacArthur, J., S. Dudley, and H.A. Williams
  2001 Approaches to facilitating health care acceptance: A case example from Karenni refugees. Pp. 56-69 in *Caring for Those in Crisis: Integrating Anthropology and Public Health in Complex Humanitarian Emergencies.* National Association for Practicing Anthropologists Bulletin, Series 21, H.A. Williams, ed. Washington, DC: American Anthropological Association.
MacCormack, C.P., R.W. Snow, and B.M. Greenwood
  1989 Use of insecticide-impregnated bed nets in Gambian primary health care: Economic aspects. *Bulletin of the World Health Organization* 67:209-214.

Mackey, L.J., I.A. McGregor, N. Paounova, and P.H. Lambert
   1982 Diagnosis of *Plasmodium falciparum* infection in man: Detection of parasite antigens by ELISA. *Bulletin of the World Health Organization* 60:69-75.
Makemba, A., P.J. Winch, S. Kamazina, V.R. Makame, F. Sengo, P.B. Lubega, J. Minjas, and C.J. Shiff
   1995 Community-based sale, distribution, and insecticide impregnation of mosquito nets in Bagamoyo District, Tanzania. *Health Policy and Planning* 10:50-59.
Makler, M.T., C.J. Palmer, and A.L. Ager
   1998 A review of practical techniques for the diagnosis of malaria. *Annals of Tropical Medicine and Parasitology* 92:419-433.
Malakooti, M.A., K. Biomndo, and G.D. Shanks
   1998 Reemergence of epidemic malaria in the highlands of western Kenya. *Emerging Infectious Diseases* 4:671-676.
Martens, P., and L. Hall
   2000 Malaria on the move: Human population movement and malaria transmission. *Emerging Infectious Diseases* 6:103-109.
Martin, A.A., J. Moore, C. Collins, R. Biellik, U. Kattel, M.J. Toole, and P.S. Moore
   1994 Infectious disease surveillance during emergency relief to Bhutanese refugees in Nepal. *Journal of the American Medical Association* 272:377-381.
Mason, J., and P. Cavalie
   1965 Malaria epidemic in Haiti following a hurricane. *American Journal of Tropical Medicine and Hygiene* 14:533-539.
McClelland, D.G., E. Adelsko, R. Hill, J. Mason, and R. Muscat
   2000 *Complex Humanitarian Emergencies and USAID's Humanitarian Response.* U.S. Agency for International Development Program and Operations Report No. 27. Washington, DC: Center for Development Information and Evaluation, U.S. Agency for International Development.
McCombie, S.C.
   1996 Treatment seeking for malaria: A review of recent research. *Social Science and Medicine* 43:933-945.
McCormick, M.C.
   1985 The contribution of low birth weight to infant mortality and childhood mortality. *New England Journal of Medicine* 312:82-90.
McFayden, J.E., ed.
   1999 *International Drug Price Indicator Guide.* Arlington, VA: Management Sciences for Health.
McGready, R., T. Cho, J.J. Cho, J.A. Simpson, C. Luxemburger, I. Dubowitz, S. Looareesuwan, N.J. White, and F. Nosten
   1998 Artemisinin derivatives in the treatment of falciparum malaria in pregnancy. *Transactions of the Royal Society of Tropical Medicine and Hygiene* 92(4):430-433.
McGready, R., A. Brockman, T. Cho, D. Cho, M. van Vugt, C. Luxemburger, T. Chongsuphajaisiddhi, N.J. White, and F. Nosten
   2000 Randomized comparison of mefloquine-artesunate versus quinine in the treatment of multidrug-resistant malaria in pregnancy. *Transactions of the Royal Society of Tropical Medicine and Hygiene* 94:689-693.

McGregor, I.A.

    1982   Malaria: Nutritional implications. *Reviews of Infectious Diseases* 4:798-804.

    1984   Epidemiology, malaria and pregnancy. *American Journal of Tropical Medicine and Hygiene* 33:517-525.

Medical Economics Co., Inc.

    1999   *Drug Topics Redbook.* Montvale, NJ: Author.

Meek, S.R.

    1989   Vector-borne diseases among displaced Kampucheans. Pp. 165-180 in *Demography and Vector-borne Diseases*, M.W. Service, ed., Boca Raton, FL: CRC Press.

Meek, S.R., M. Rowland, and M. Connolly

    1999   *WHO/RBM, WHO/Emergency and Humanitarian Action: Outline Strategy for Malaria Control in Complex Emergencies.* Geneva: World Health Organization.

Menendez, C., J. Todd, P.L. Alonso, N. Francis, S. Lulat, S. Ceesay, B. M'Boge, and B.M. Greenwood

    1994   The effects of iron supplementation during pregnancy, given by traditional birth attendants, on the prevalence of anaemia and malaria. *Transactions of the Royal Society of Tropical Medicine and Hygiene* 88(5):590-593.

Menendez, C., E. Kahigwa, R. Hirt, P. Vounatsou, J.J. Aponte, F. Font, C.J. Acosta, D.M. Schellenberg, C.M. Galindo, J. Kimario, H. Urassa, B. Brabin, T.A. Smith, A.Y. Kitua, M. Tanner, and P.L. Alonso

    1997   Randomised, placebo-controlled trial of iron supplementation and malaria chemoprophylaxis for prevention of severe anaemia and malaria in Tanzanian infants. *Lancet* 350(9081):844-850.

Miller, K.D., H.O. Lobel, R.F. Satriale, J.N. Kuritsky, R. Stern, and C.C. Campbell

    1986   Severe cutaneous reactions among American travelers using pyrimethamine-sulfadoxine (Fansidar) for malaria prophylaxis. *American Journal of Tropical Medicine and Hygiene* 35:451-458.

Miller, L.H., F.M. McAuliffe, and S.J. Mason

    1977   Erythrocyte receptors for malaria merozoites. *American Journal of Tropical Medicine and Hygiene* 26:204-208.

Mockenhaupt, F.P.

    1995   Mefloquine resistance in *Plasmodium falciparum. Parasitology Today* 11:248-253.

Molyneux, M.E., T.E. Taylor, J.J. Wirima, and J. Borgstein

    1989   Clinical features and prognostic indicators in paediatric cerebral malaria: A study of 131 comatose Malawian children. *Quarterly Journal of Medicine* 71:441-459.

Monlun, E., P. Le Metayer, S. Szwandt, D. Neau, M. Longy-Boursier, and J. Horton

    1995   Cardiac complications of halofantrine: A prospective study of 20 patients. *Transactions of the Royal Society of Tropical Medicine and Hygiene* 89:430-433.

Moody, A.

    2002   Rapid diagnostic tests for malaria parasites. *Clinical Microbiology Reviews* 15(1):66-78 (January).

Mouchet, J., S. Manguin, J. Sircoulon, S. Laventure, O. Faye, A.W. Onapa, P. Carnevale, J. Julvez, and D. Fontenille

    1998   Evolution of malaria in Africa for the past 40 years: Impact of climatic and human factors. *Journal of the American Mosquito Control Association* 14:121-130.

Muhe, L., B. Oljira, H. Degefu, S. Jaffar, and M.W. Weber
  2000 Evaluation of clinical pallor in the identification and treatment of children with moderate and severe anemia. *Tropical Medicine and International Health* 5:805-810.
Murphy, G.S., H. Basri, Purnomo, E.M. Anderson, M.J. Bangs, D.L. Mount, J. Gorden, A.A. Lal, A.R. Purwokusumo, S. Harjosuwarno, K. Sorensen, and S.L. Hoffman
  1993 Vivax malaria resistant to treatment and prophylaxis with chloroquine. *Lancet* 341(8837):96-100.
Murray, M.J., A.B. Murray, M.B. Murray, and C.J. Murray
  1976 Somali food shelters in the Ogaden famine and their impact on health. *Lancet* (7972):1283-1285.
  1977 The adverse effect of iron repletion on the course of certain infections. *British Medical Journal* 2(6145):1113-1114.
Murray, M.J., A.B. Murray, N.J. Murray, and M.B. Murray
  1978 Diet and cerebral malaria: The effect of famine and refeeding. *American Journal of Clinical Nutrition* 31(1):57-61.
Mutabingwa, T., A. Nzila, E. Mberu, E. Nduati, P. Winstanley, E. Hills, and W. Watkins
  2001 Chlorproguanil-dapsone for treatment of drug-resistant falciparum malaria in Tanzania. *Lancet* 358:1218-1223.
Nichter, M.
  1999 Project community diagnosis: Participatory research as a first-step toward community involvement in primary health care. Pp. 300-324 in *Anthropology in Public Health: Bridging Differences in Culture and Society*, R. Hahn, ed. New York: Oxford University Press.
Nosten, F., F. ter Kuile, L. Maelankirri, B. Decludt, and N.J. White
  1991 Malaria during pregnancy in an area of unstable endemicity. *Transactions of the Royal Society of Tropical Medicine & Hygiene* 85:424-429.
Nosten, F., F.O. ter Kuile, C. Luxemburger, C. Woodrow, D.E. Kyle, T. Chongsuphajaisiddhi, and N.J. White
  1993 Cardiac effects of antimalarial treatment with halofantrine. *Lancet* 341(8852):1054-1056.
Nosten, F., C. Luxemburger, F.O. ter Kuile, C. Woodrow, J.P. Eh, and N.J. White
  1994a Treatment of multidrug-resistant *Plasmodium falciparum* malaria with 3-day artesunate-mefloquine combination. *Journal of Infectious Diseases* 170:971-977.
Nosten, F., F. ter Kuile, L. Maelankiri L., T. Chongsuphajaisiddhi, L. Nopdonrattakoon, S. Tangkitchot, E. Boudreau, D. Bunnag, and N.J. White
  1994b Mefloquine prophylaxis prevents malaria during pregnancy: A double-blind, placebo-controlled study. *Journal of Infectious Diseases* 169(3):595-603.
Nosten, F., R. McGready, J.A. Simpson, K.L. Thwai, S. Balkan, T. Cho, L. Hkirijaroen, S. Looareesuwan, and N.J. White
  1999a Effects of *Plasmodium vivax* malaria in pregnancy. *Lancet* 354:546-549.
Nosten, F., M. Vincenti, J. Simpson, P. Yei, K.L. Thwai, J. Pa Eh, T. Chongsuphajaisiddhi, and N.J. White
  1999b The effects of mefloquine treatment in pregnancy. *Clinical Infectious Diseases* 28:808-815.

Nosten, F., M. van Vugt, R. Price, C. Luxemburger, K.L. Thway, A. Brockman, R. McGready, F. ter Kuile, S. Looareesuwan, and N.J. White
    2000   Effects of artesunate-mefloquine combination on incidence of *Plasmodium falciparum* malaria and mefloquine resistance in western Thailand: A prospective study. *Lancet* 356(9226):297-302.

Obonyo, C.O., E.W. Steyerberg, A.J. Oloo, and D.F. Habbema
    1998   Blood transfusions for severe malaria-related anemia in Africa: A decision analysis. *American Journal of Tropical Medicine and Hygiene* 59:808-812.

Olivar, M., M. Develoux, A. Chegou Abari, and L. Loutan
    1991   Presumptive diagnosis of malaria results in a significant risk of mistreatment of children in urban Sahel. *Transactions of the Royal Society of Tropical Medicine and Hygiene* 85:729-730.

Olliaro, P., J. Cattani, and D. Wirth
    1996   Malaria, the submerged disease. *Journal of the American Medical Association* 275:230-233.

Oppenheimer, S.J., F.D. Gibson, S.B. Macfarlane, J.B. Moody, C. Harrison, A. Spencer, and O. Bunari
    1986a Iron supplementation increases prevalence and effects of malaria: Report on clinical studies in Papua New Guinea. *Transactions of the Royal Society of Tropical Medicine and Hygiene* 80(4):603-612.

Oppenheimer, S.J., S.B. Macfarlane, J.B. Moody, and C. Harrison
    1986b Total dose iron infusion, malaria and pregnancy in Papua New Guinea. *Transactions of the Royal Society of Tropical Medicine and Hygiene* 80:818-822.

Palmer, C.A., and A. Zwi
    1998   Women, health and humanitarian aid in conflict. *Disasters* 22:236-249.

Palmer, C.A., L. Lush, and A. Zwi
    1999   The emerging international policy agenda for reproductive health services in conflict settings. *Social Science and Medicine* 49:1689-1703.

Palmer, C.J., L. Validum, J. Lindo, A. Campa, C. Validum, M. Makler, R.R. Cuadrado, and A. Ager
    1999   Field evaluation of the OptiMAL rapid malaria diagnostic test during anti-malarial therapy in Guyana. *Transactions of the Royal Society of Tropical Medicine and Hygiene* 93(5):517-518.

Pan American Health Organization
    1995   Regional status of malaria in the Americas, 1994. *Epidemiologic Bulletin* 16:10-14.

Parise, M.E., J.G. Ayisi, B.L. Nahlen, L.J. Schlultz, J.M. Roberts, A. Misore, R. Muga, A.J. Oloo, and R.W. Steketee
    1998   Efficacy of sulfadoxine-pyrimethamine for prevention of placental malaria in an area of Kenya with a high prevalence of malaria and human immunodeficiency virus infection. *American Journal of Tropical Medicine and Hygiene* 59:813-822.

Parola, P., S. Ranque, S. Badiaga, M. Niang, O. Blin, J.J. Charbit, J. Delmont, and P. Brouqui
    2001   Controlled trial of 3-day quinine-clindamycin treatment versus 7-day quinine treatment for adult travelers with uncomplicated falciparum malaria imported from the Tropics. *Antimicrobial Agents and Chemotherapy* 45:932-935.

PATH

1997 *Anemia Detection Methods in Low-Resource Settings: A Manual for Health Workers.* Seattle, WA: Program for Appropriate Technology in Health.

Paxton, L.A., L. Slutsker, L.J. Schultz, S.P. Luby, R. Meriwether, P. Matson, and A.J. Sulzer

1996 Imported malaria in Montagnard refugees settling in North Carolina: Implications for prevention and control. *American Journal of Tropical Medicine and Hygiene* 54:54-57.

Perkins, B.A., J.R. Zucker, J. Otieno, H.S. Jafari, L. Paxton, S.C. Redd, B.L. Nahlen, B. Schwartz, A.J. Oloo, C. Olango, S. Gove, and C.C. Campbell

1997 Evaluation of an alogrithm for integrated management of childhood illness in an area of Kenya with high malaria transmission. *Bulletin of the World Health Organization* 75(Suppl. 1):33-42.

Peterson, E.A., L. Roberts, M.J. Toole, and D.E. Peterson

1998 The effect of soap distribution on diarrhoea: Nyamithuthu refugee camp. *International Journal of Epidemiology* 27:520-524.

Phillips-Howard, P.A.

1999 Epidemiological and control issues related to malaria in pregnancy. *Annals of Tropical Medicine and Parasitology* 93(Suppl. 1):S11-S17.

Piper, R., J. LeBras, L. Wentworth, A. Hunt-Cooke, S. Houze, P. Chiodini, and M. Makler

1999 Immunocapture diagnostic assays for malaria using *Plasmodium* lactate dehydrogenase (pLDH). *American Journal of Tropical Medicine and Hygiene* 60(1):109-118.

Pitt, S., B.E. Pearcy, R.H. Stevens, A. Sharipov, K. Satarov, and N. Banatvala

1998 War in Tajikistan and re-emergence of *Plasmodium falciparum. Lancet* 352:1279.

Plowe, C.V., A. Djimdé, M. Bouare, O. Doumbo, and T.E. Wellems

1995 Pyrimethamine and proguanil resistance-conferring mutations in *Plasmodium falciparum* dihydrofolate reductase: Polymerase chain reaction methods for surveillance in Africa. *American Journal of Tropical Medicine and Hygiene* 52:565-568.

Price, R.N., F. Nosten, C. Luxemburger, F.O. ter Kuile, L. Paiphun, T. Chongsuphajaisiddhi, and N.J. White

1996 Effects of artemisinin derivatives on malaria transmissibility. *Lancet* 347(9016): 1654-1658.

Price, R.N., F. Nosten, C. Luxemburger, M. van Vugt, L. Phaipun, T. Chongsuphajaisiddhi, and N.J. White

1997 Artesunate/mefloquine treatment of multi-drug resistant falciparum malaria. *Transactions of the Royal Society of Tropical Medicine and Hygiene* 91:574-577.

Prothero, R.M.

1977 Disease and mobility: A neglected factor in epidemiology. *International Journal of Epidemiology* 6:259-267.

1989 Problems of human mobility and diseases. Pp. 1-16 in *Demography and Vector-borne Diseases,* M.W. Service, ed. Boca Raton, FL: CRC Press.

1994 Forced movements of population and health hazards in tropical Africa. *International Journal of Epidemiology* 23:657-664.

Pukrittayakamee, S., A. Chantra, J.A. Simpson, S. Vanijanonta, Clemens, S. Looaresssuwan, and N.J. White
  2000a Therapeutic responses to different antimalarial drugs in vivax malaria. *Antimicrobial Agents and Chemotherapy* 44:1680-1685.

Pukrittayakamee, S., A. Chantra, S. Vanijanonta, R. Clemens, S. Looareesuwan, and N.J. White
  2000b Therapeutic responses to quinine and clindamycin in multidrug-resistant falciparum malaria. *Antimicrobial Agents and Chemotherapy* 44:2395-2398.

Radloff, P.D., J. Phillipps, M. Nkeyi, D. Hutchinson, and P.G. Kremsner
  1996 Atovaquone and proguanil for *Plasmodium falciparum* malaria. *Lancet* 347:1511-1513.

Redd, S.C., P.B. Bloland, P.N. Kazembe, E. Patrick, R. Tembenu, and C.C. Campbell
  1992 Usefulness of clinical case definitions in guiding therapy for African children with malaria or pneumonia. *Lancet* 340(8828):1140-1143.

Rey, J.L., J.D. Cavallo, J.M. Milleliri, S. L'Hoest, J.L. Soares, N. Piny, J.C. Coue, and A. Jouan
  1996 Fever of unknown origin (FUO) in the camps of Rwandan refugees in the Goma region of Zaire. *Bulletin de la Societe de Pathologie Exotique* 89:204-208.

Rickman, L.S., G.W. Long, R. Oberst, A. Cabanban, R. Sangalang, J.I. Smith, J.D. Chulay, and S.L. Hoffman
  1989 Rapid diagnosis of malaria by acridine orange staining of centrifuged parasites. *Lancet* (8628):68-71.

Ringwald, P., J. Bickii, and L. Basco
  1996 Randomised trial of pyronaridine versus chloroquine for acute uncomplicated falciparum malaria in Africa. *Lancet* 347:24-27.

Robb, A.
  1999 Malaria and pregnancy: The implementation of interventions. *Annals of Tropical Medicine and Parasitology* 93(Suppl. 1):S67-S70.

Romi, R., B. Ravoniharimelina, M. Ramiakajato, and G. Majori
  1993 Field trials of *Bacillus thuringiensis* H-14 and *Bacillus sphaericus* (strain 2362) formulations against *Anopheles arabiensis* in the central highlands of Madagascar. *Journal of the American Mosquito Control Association* 9:325-329.

Roundy, R.W.
  1976 Altitudinal mobility and disease hazards for Ethiopian populations. *Economic Geography* 52:103-115.

Rowland M.
  1999 Malaria control: Bednets or spraying? Malaria control in the Afghan refugee camps of western Pakistan. *Transactions of the Royal Society of Tropical Medicine and Hygiene* 93:458-459.

  2001 Malaria control in Afghan refugee camps: Novel solutions. *Transactions of the Royal Society of Tropical Medicine and Hygiene* 95:125-126.

Rowland, M., and N. Durrani
  1999 Randomized controlled trials of 5- and 14-days primaquine therapy against relapses of vivax malaria in an Afghan refugee settlement in Pakistan. *Transactions of the Royal Society of Tropical Medicine and Hygiene* 93:641-643.

Rowland, M., and F. Nosten
  2001 Malaria epidemiology and control in refugee camps and complex emergencies. *Annals of Tropical Medicine and Parasitology* 95:741-754.
Rowland, M., M. Bouma, D. Ducornez, N. Durrani, J. Rozendaal, A. Schapira, and E. Sondorp
  1996 Pyrethroid-impregnated bed nets for personal protection against malaria for Afghan refugees. *Transactions of the Royal Society of Tropical Medicine and Hygiene* 90:357-361.
Rowland, M., N. Durrani, S. Hewitt, N. Mohammed, M. Bouma, I. Carneiro, J. Rozendaal, and A. Schapira
  1999 Permethrin-treated chaddars and top-sheets: Appropriate technology for protection against malaria in Afghanistan and other complex emergencies. *Transactions of the Royal Society of Tropical Medicine and Hygiene* 93:465-472.
Sáenz, R., R.A. Bissell, and F. Paniagua
  1995 Post-disaster malaria in Costa Rica. *Prehospital and Disaster Medicine* 10:154-160.
Sahr, F., V.R. Willoughby, A.A. Gbakima, and M.J. Bockarie
  2001 Apparent drug failure following artesunate treatment of *Plasmodium falciparum* malaria in Freetown, Sierra Leone: Four case reports. *Annals of Tropical Medicine and Parasitology* 95:445-459.
Salako, L.A., O. Walker, A. Sowunmi, S.J. Omokhodion, R. Adio, and A.M. Oduola
  1994 Artemether in moderately severe and cerebral malaria in Nigerian children. *Transactions of the Royal Society of Tropical Medicine and Hygiene* 88(Suppl. 1):S13-S15.
Salama, P., F. Assefa, L. Talley, P. Spiegel, A. van der Veen, and C. Gotway
  2001 Malnutrition, measles, mortality, and the humanitarian response during a famine in Ethiopia. *Journal of the American Medical Association* 286:563-571.
Sawyer, D.
  1993 Economic and social consequences of malaria in new colonization projects in Brazil. *Social Science and Medicine* 37:1131-1136.
Schellenberg, D., C. Menendez, E. Kahigwa, J. Aponte, J. Vidal, M. Tanner, H. Mshinda, and P. Alonso
  2001 Intermittent treatment for malaria and anemia control at time of routine vaccinations in Tanzanian infants: A randomized, placebo-controlled trial. *Lancet* 357:1471-1477.
Schultz, L.J., R.W. Steketee, A. Macheso, P. Kazembe, L. Chitsulo, and J.J. Wirima
  1994 The efficacy of antimalarial regimens containing sylfadoxine/pyrimethamine and/or chloroquine in preventing peripheral and placental *Plasmodium falciparum* infection among pregnant women in Malawi. *American Journal of Tropical Medicine and Hygiene* 51:515-522.
Schultz, L.J., R.W. Steketee, L. Chitsulo, and J.J. Wirima
  1995 Antimalarials during pregnancy: A cost-effectiveness analysis. *Bulletin of the World Health Organization* 73:207-214.
Seaman, J.
  1999 Malnutrition in emergencies: How can we do better and where do the responsibilities lie? *Disasters* 23:306-315.

Service, M.W.

1990 *Livestock Management and Disease Vector Control.* Report of the 10th Meeting of the Panel of Experts on Environmental Management for Vector Control (WHO/CWS/91.11) Geneva: World Health Organization.

1993 The *Anopheles* vector. Pp. 96-123 in *Bruce-Chwatt's Essential Malariology*, 3rd ed. H.M. Gilles and D.A. Warrell, eds. New York: Oxford University Press.

Shankar, A.H.

2000 Nutritional modulation of malaria morbidity and mortality. *Journal of Infectious Diseases* 182(Suppl. 1):S37-S53.

Shankar, A.H., B. Genton, M. Baisor, J. Paino, S. Tamja, T. Adiguma, L. Wu, L. Rare, D. Bannon, J.M. Tielsch, K.P. West Jr., and M.P. Alpers

2000 The influence of zinc supplementation on morbidity due to *Plasmodium falciparum*: A randomized trial in pre-school children in Papua New Guinea. *American Journal of Tropical Medicine and Hygiene* 62:633-639.

Shanks, G.D., K. Biomndo, S.I. Hay, and R.W. Snow

2000 Changing patterns of clinical malaria since 1965 among a tea estate population located in the Kenyan highlands. *Transactions of the Royal Society of Tropical Medicine and Hygiene* 94:253-255.

Sharp, T.W., F.M. Burkle, A.F. Vaughn, R. Chotani, and R.J. Brennan

2002 Challenges and opportunities for humanitarian relief in Afghanistan. *Clinical Infectious Diseases* 34(Suppl.):S215-S228.

Shulman, C.E., E.K. Dorman, F. Cutts, K. Kawuondo, J.N. Bulmer, N. Peshu, and K. Marsh

1999 Intermittent sulphadoxine-pyrimethamine to prevent severe anemia secondary to malaria in pregnancy: A randomized placebo-controlled trial. *Lancet* 353:632-636.

Sibley, C.H., J.E. Hyde, P.F. Sims, C.V. Plowe, J.G. Kublin, E.K. Mberu, A.F. Cowman, P.A. Winstanley, W.M. Watkins, and A.M. Nzila

2001 Pyrimethamine-sulfadoxine resistance in *Plasmodium falciparum*: What next? *Trends in Parasitology* 17(12):582-588.

Singh, N., R.K. Mehra, and V.P. Sharma

1999 Malaria and the Narmada River development in India: A case study of the Bargi Dam. *Annals of Tropical Medicine and Parasitology* 93:477-488.

Singhanetra-Renard, A.

1993 Malaria and mobility in Thailand. *Social Science and Medicine* 37(9):1147-1154.

Singhasivanon, P.

1999 Mekong malaria: Malaria, multidrug resistance and economic development in the greater Mekong subregion of Southeast Asia. *Southeast Asian Journal of Tropical Medicine and Public Health* 30(Suppl. 4):1-101.

Slutsker, L., T.E. Taylor, J.J. Wirima, and R.W. Steketee

1994 In-hospital morbidity and mortality due to malaria-associated severe anaemia in two areas of Malawi with different patterns of malaria infection. *Transactions of the Royal Society of Tropical Medicine and Hygiene* 88:548-551.

Slutsker, L., M. Tipple, V. Keane, C. McCance, and C.C. Campbell

1995 Malaria in East African refugees resettling to the United States: Development of strategies to reduce the risk of imported malaria. *Journal of Infectious Diseases* 171:489-493.

Smith, A.W., R.G. Hendrickse, C. Harrison, R.J. Hayes, and B.M. Greenwood
  1989 The effects on malaria of treatment of iron-deficiency anaemia with oral iron in Gambian children. *Annals of Tropical Paediatrics* 9:17-23.
Smith, T., J. Armstrong Schellenberg, J.R. Armstrong Schellenberg, and R. Hayes
  1994 Attributable fraction estimates and case definitions for malaria in endemic areas. *Statistics in Medicine* 13:2345-2358.
Snow, R.W., P. Byass, F.C. Shenton, and B.M. Greenwood
  1991 The relationship between anthropometric measurements and measurements of iron status and susceptibility to malaria in Gambian children. *Transactions of the Royal Society of Tropical Medicine and Hygiene* 85:584-589.
Snow, R.W., I. Bastos de Azevedo, B.S. Lowe, E.W. Kabiru, C.G. Nevill, S. Mwankusye, G. Kassiga, K. Marsh, and T. Teuscher
  1994 Severe childhood malaria in two areas of markedly different falciparum transmission in East Africa. *Acta Tropica* 57(4):289-300.
Snow, R.W., M. Craig, U. Deichmann, and K. Marsh
  1999 Estimating mortality, morbidity and disability due to malaria among Africa's non-pregnant population. *Bulletin of the World Health Organization* 77:624-640.
Sowunmi, A., and J.A. Akindele
  1993 Presumptive diagnosis of malaria in infants in an endemic area. *Transactions of the Royal Society of Tropical Medicine and Hygiene* 87:422.
Sphere Project
  2000 *Humanitarian Charter and Minimum Standards in Disaster Response.* Oxford: Oxford Publishing.
Spiegel, P., and P. Salama
  2000 War and mortality in Kosovo, 1998-99: An epidemiological testimony. *Lancet* 355:2204-2209.
  2001 Emergencies in developed countries: Are aid organizations ready to adapt? *Lancet* 357:714.
Steffen, R., E. Fuchs, J. Schildknecht, U. Naef, M. Funk, P. Schlagenhauf, P. Phillips-Howard, C. Nevill, and D. Stürchler
  1993 Mefloquine compared with other malaria chemoprophylactic regimens in tourists visiting East Africa. *Lancet* 341:1299-1303.
Steketee, R.W., J.J. Wirima, and C.C. Campbell
  1996a Developing effective strategies for malaria prevention programs for pregnant African women. *American Journal of Tropical Medicine and Hygiene* 55(Suppl. 1):95-100.
Steketee, R.W., J.J. Wirima, P.B. Bloland, B. Chilima, J.H. Mermin, and L. Chitsulo
  1996b Impairment of a pregnant woman's acquired ability to limit *Plasmodium falciparum* by infection with human immunodeficiency virus type-1. *American Journal of Tropical Medicine and Hygiene* 55(Suppl. 1):42-49.
Steketee, R.W., J.J. Wirima, L. Slutsker, D.L. Heymann, and J.G. Breman
  1996c The problem of malaria and malaria control in pregnancy in sub-Saharan Africa. *American Journal of Tropical Medicine and Hygiene* 55(Suppl. 1):2-7.
Stott, G.J., and S.M. Lewis
  1995 A simple and reliable method for estimating haemoglobin. *Bulletin of the World Health Organization* 73(3):369-373.

Suleman, M.
  1988   Malaria in Afghan refugees in Pakistan. *Transactions of the Royal Society of Tropical Medicine and Hygiene* 82:44-47.
Taylor, T.E., B.A. Wills, P. Kazembe, M. Chisale, J.J. Wirima, E.Y. Ratsma, and M.E. Molyneux
  1993   Rapid coma resolution with artemether in Malawian children with cerebral malaria. *Lancet* 341(8846):661-662.
Teklehaimanot, A.
  1986   Chloroquine-resistant *Plasmodium falciparum* malaria in Ethiopia. *Lancet* 2:127-129.
ter Kuile, F.O., G. Dolan, F. Nosten, M.D. Edstein, C. Luxemburger, L. Phaipun, T. Chongsuphajaisiddhi, H.K. Webster, and N.J. White
  1993   Halofantrine versus mefloquine in treatment of multidrug-resistant falciparum malaria. *Lancet* 341(8852):1044-1049.
Thaithong, S., L. Suebsaeng, W. Rooney, and G.H. Beale
  1988   Evidence of increased chloroquine sensitivity in Thai isolates of *Plasmodium falciparum*. *Transactions of the Royal Society of Tropical Medicine and Hygiene* 82:37-38.
Tharavanij, S.
  1990   New developments in malaria diagnostic techniques. *Southeast Asian Journal of Tropical Medicine and Public Health* 21:3-16.
Thimasarn, K., J. Sirichaisinthop, S. Vijaykadga, S. Tansophalaks, P. Yamokgul, A. Laomiphol, C. Palananth, U. Thamewat, S. Thaithong, and W. Rooney
  1995   In vivo study of the response of *Plasmodium falciparum* to standard mefloquine/sulfadoxine/pyrimethamine (MSP) treatment among gem miners returning from Cambodia. *Southeast Asian Journal of Tropical Medicine and Public Health* 26(2):204-212.
Tomashek, K.M., B.A. Woodruff, C.A. Gotway, P. Bloland, and G. Mbaruku
  2001   Randomized intervention study comparing several regimens for the treatment of moderate anemia among refugee children in Kigoma region, Tanzania. *American Journal of Tropical Medicine and Hygiene* 64:164-171.
Toole, M.J., and R.J. Waldman
  1988   An analysis of mortality trends among refugee populations in Somalia, Sudan, and Thailand. *Bulletin of the World Health Organization* 66(2):237-247.
  1990   Prevention of excess mortality in refugee and displaced populations in developing countries. *Journal of the American Medical Association* 263:3296-3302.
  1993   Refugees and displaced persons. War, hunger, and public health. *Journal of the American Medical Association* 270:600-605.
U.S. Committee for Refugees
  2000   *World Refugee Survey 2000*. Washington, DC: Immigration and Refugee Services of America.
Van Bortel, W., M. Barutwanayo, C. Delacollette, and M. Coosemans
  1996   Motivation to acquire and use impregnated mosquito nets in a stable malaria zone in Burundi. *Tropical Medicine and International Health* 1(1):71-80.

Van Damme, W., V. De Brouwere, M. Boelaert, and W. Van Lerbergh
    1998   Effects of a refugee-assistance programme on host population in Guinea as measured by obstetric interventions. *Lancet* 351:1609-1613.
van der Geest, S.
    1997   Is there a role for traditional medicine in basic health services in Africa? A plea for a community perspective. *Tropical Medicine and International Health* 2:903-911.
van Hensbroek, M.B., S. Morris-Jones, S. Meisner, S. Jaffar, L. Bayo, R. Dackour, C. Phillips, and B.M. Greenwood
    1995   Iron, but not folic acid, combined with effective antimalarial therapy promotes haematological recovery in African children after acute falciparum malaria. *Transactions of the Royal Society of Tropical Medicine and Hygiene* 89(6):672-676.
van Vugt, M., F. Ezzet, F. Nosten, I. Gathmann, P. Wilairatana, S. Looareesuwan, and N.J. White
    1999   No evidence of cardiotoxicity during antimalarial treatment with artemether-lumefantrine. *American Journal of Tropical Medicine and Hygiene* 61:964-967.
van Vugt, M., S. Looareesuwan, P. Wilairatana, R. McGreedy, L. Villegas, I. Gathmann, R. Mull, A. Brockman, N.J. White, and F. Nosten
    2000   Artemether-lumefantrine for the treatment of multi-drug resistant falciparum malaria. *Transactions of the Royal Society of Tropical Medicine and Hygiene* 94:545-548.
Veeken, H.
    1993   Malaria and gold fever. *British Medical Journal* 307:433-434.
Verdrager, J.
    1986   Epidemiology of the emergence and spread of drug-resistant falciparum malaria in South-east Asia and Australasia. *Journal of Tropical Medicine and Hygiene* 89:277-289.
Verhoeff, F.H., B.J. Brabin, L. Chimsuku, P. Kazembe, W.B. Russell, and R.L. Broadhead
    1997   An evaluation of the effects of intermittent sulfadoxine-pyrimethamine treatment in pregnancy on parasite clearance and risk of low birthweight in rural Malawi. *Annals of Tropical Medicine and Parasitology* 92:141-150.
von Seidlein L., P. Milligan, M. Pinder, K. Bojang, C. Anyalebechi, R. Gosling, R. Coleman, J.L. Ude, A. Sadiq, M. Duraisingh, D. Warhurst, A. Alloueche, G. Targett, K. McAdam, B. Greenwood, G. Walraven, P. Olliaro, and T. Doherty
    2000   Efficacy of artesuante plus pyrimethamine-sulphadoxine for uncomplicated malaria in Gambian children: A double-blind, randomized, controlled trial. *Lancet* 355(9220):352-357.
Waldman, R.J.
    2001   Prioritising health care in complex emergencies. *Lancet* 357:1427-1429.
Waldman, R., and G. Martone
    1999   Public health and complex emergencies: New issues, new conditions. *American Journal of Public Health* 89:1483-1485.
Waldman, R., and H.A. Williams
    2001   Public health in complex emergencies: Toward a more integrated science. Pp. 89-111 in *Caring for Those in Crisis: Integrating Anthropology and Public Health in Complex Humanitarian Emergencies*. National Association for Practicing Anthropologists Bulletin Series 21, H.A. Williams, ed. Washington, DC: American Anthropological Association.

Walkup, M.

1997   Policy dysfunction in humanitarian organizations: The role of coping strategies, institutions, and organizational culture. *Journal of Refugee Studies* 10:37-60.

Walsh, D.S., S. Looareesuwan, P. Wilairatana, D.G. Heppner, D.B. Tang, T.G. Brewer, W. Chokejindachai, P. Viriyavejakul, D.E. Kyle, W.K. Milhous, B.G. Schuster, J. Horton, D.J. Braitman, and R.P. Brueckner

1999   Randomized dose-ranging study of the safety and efficacy of WR238605 (Tafenoquine) in the prevention of relapse of *Plasmodium vivax* malaria in Thailand. *Journal of Infectious Diseases* 180(4):1282-1287.

Watkins, W.M., E.K. Mberu, P.A. Winstanley, and C.V. Plowe

1997   The efficacy of antifolate antimalarial combinations in Africa: A predictive model based on pharmacodynamic and pharmacokinetic analyses. *Parasitology Today* 13:459-464.

Webb, P., and A. Harinarayan

1999   A measure of uncertainty: The nature of vulnerability and its relationship to malnutrition. *Disasters* 23:292-305.

Weber, M.W., E.K. Mulholland, S. Jaffar, H. Troedsson, S. Gove, and B.M. Greenwood

1996   Evaluation of an algorithm for the integrated management of childhood illness in an area with seasonal malaria in the Gambia. *Bulletin of the World Health Organization* 75(Suppl. 1):25-32.

Weiss, W.M., and P. Bolton

2000   *Training in Qualitative Research Methods for PVOs and NGOs (and counterparts): A Trainer's Guide to Strengthen Program Planning and Evaluation.* Baltimore, MD: The Johns Hopkins University School of Public Health, Center for Refugee and Disaster Studies. Also available: <*http://www.jhsph.edu/refugee/images/tqr_a_docs/ tg_introduction.pdf*>.

White, N.

1999   Antimalarial drug resistance and mortality in falciparum malaria. *Tropical Medicine and International Health* 4:469-470.

White, N.J., F. Nosten, S. Looareesuwan, W.M. Watkins, K. Marsh, R.W. Snow, G. Kokwaro, J. Ouma, TT. Hien, M.E. Molyneux, T.E. Taylor, C.I. Newbold, T.K. Ruebush II, M. Danis, B.M. Greenwood, R.M. Anderson, and P. Olliaro

1999   Averting a malaria disaster. *Lancet* 353(9168):1965-1967.

Whitworth, J., D. Morgan, M. Quigley, A. Smith, B. Mayanja, H. Eotu, N. Omoding, M. Okongo, S. Malamba, and A. Ojwiya

2000   Effect of HIV-1 and increasing immunosuppression on malaria parasitaemia and clinical episodes in adults in rural Uganda: A cohort study. *Lancet* 356(9235): 1051-1056.

Whyte, B.

2000   News item. *Bulletin of the World Health Organization* 78:1062.

Williams, H.A., and P.B. Bloland

2001   A practical discussion of applied public health research in the context of complex emergencies: Examples from malaria control in refugee camps. Pp. 70-88 in *Caring for Those in Crisis: Integrating Anthropology and Public Health in Complex Humanitarian Emergencies.* National Association for Practicing Anthropologists Bulletin Series 21, H.A. Williams, ed. Washington, DC: American Anthropological Association.

Williams, H.A., S.P. Kachur, N.C. Nalwamba, A. Hightower, C. Simoonga, and P.C. Mphande
  1999 A community perspective on the efficacy of malaria treatment options for children in Lundazi District, Zambia. *Tropical Medicine and International Health* 4:641-652.
Williams, T.N., K. Maitland, L. Phelps, S. Bennett, T.E.A. Peto, J. Viji, R. Timothy, J.B. Clegg, D.J. Weatherall, and D.K. Bowden
  1997 *Plasmodium vivax:* A cause of malnutrition in young children. *Quarterly Journal of Medicine* 90:751-757.
Wilson, K.B.
  1992 Enhancing refugees' own food acquisition strategies. *Journal of Refugee Studies* 5:226-246.
Winch, P.
  1999 Anthropological methods in a mosquito net intervention. Pp. 44-62 in *Anthropology in Public Health: Bridging Differences in Culture and Society*, R.A. Hahn, ed. New York: Oxford University Press.
Winch, P.J., A.M. Makemba, D.R. Kamazima, M. Lurie, G.K. Lwihula, Z. Premji, J.N. Minjas, and C. Shiff
  1996 Local terminology for febrile illnesses in Bagamoyo District, Tanzania and its impact on the design of a community-based malaria control programme. *Social Science and Medicine* 42:1057-1067.
Winstanley, P.A.
  2000 Chemotherapy for falciparum malaria: The armoury, the problems and the prospects. *Parasitology Today* 16:146-153.
Wolday, D., T. Kibreab, D. Bukenya, and R. Hodes
  1995 Sensitivity of *Plasmodium falciparum* in vivo to chloroquine and pyrimethamine-sulfadoxine in Rwandan patients in a refugee camp in Zaire. *Transactions of the Royal Society of Tropical Medicine and Hygiene* 89:654-656.
Wolff, C.G., D.G. Schroeder, and M.W. Young
  2001 Effect of improved housing on illness in children under 5 in northern Malawi. *British Medical Journal* 322:1209-1212.
Wongsrichanalai, C., H.K. Webster, T. Wimonwattrawatee, P. Sookto, N. Chuanak, K. Thimasarn, and W.H. Wernsdorfer
  1992 Emergence of multidrug-resistant *Plasmodium falciparum* in Thailand: In vitro tracking. *American Journal of Tropical Medicine and Hygiene* 47(1):112-116.
Wongsrichanalai, C., T. Wimonwattrawatee, P. Sookto, A. Laboonchai, D.G. Heppner, D.E. Kyle, and W.H. Wernsdorfer
  1999 In vitro sensitivity of *Plasmodium falciparum* to artesunate in Thailand. *Bulletin of the World Health Organization* 77:392-398.
Wongsrichanalai, C., K. Thimasarn, and J. Sirichaisinthop
  2000 Antimalarial drug combination policy: A caveat. *Lancet* 355:2245-2247.
Wongsrichanalai, C., A.L. Pickard, W.H. Wernsdorfer, and S.R. Meshnick
  2002 Epidemiology of drug-resistant malaria. *The Lancet Infectious Diseases* 2(4):209-218.
World Health Organization
  1996a World malaria situation in 1993, part I. *Weekly Epidemiological Record* 71:17-22.

1996b A rapid dipstick antigen capture assay for the diagnosis of falciparum malaria. WHO informal consultation on recent advances in diagnostic techniques and vaccines for malaria. *Bulletin of the World Health Organization* 74:47-54.

1996c *Assessment of Therapeutic Efficacy of Antimalarial Drugs for Uncomplicated Falciparum Malaria in Areas with Intense Transmission.* (WHO/MAL/96.1077) Geneva and Brazzaville: World Health Organization.

1997a *Integrated Management of Childhood Illnesses Adaptation Guide. Part 2. C. Technical Basis for Adapting Clinical Guidelines, Feeding Recommendations, and Local Terms.* Pp. 49-51 in working draft version 3. Geneva: World Health Organization, Division of Child Health and Development.

1997b *Report of Consultation on Applied Health Research Priorities in Complex Emergencies.* WHO Headquarters, Geneva, October 28-29, 1997. Geneva: World Health Organization.

1997c *Guidelines on the Use of Insecticide-Treated Mosquito Nets for the Prevention and Control of Malaria in Africa.* (CTD/MAL/AFRO/97.4) Geneva: World Health Organization.

1998 *WHO Expert Committee on Malaria: Twentieth Report.* WHO Technical Report Series 892. Geneva: World Health Organization.

1999a *Draft Guideline Specifications for Bacterial Larvicides for Public Health Use.* Report of the WHO Informal Consultation, April 28-30, 1999. (WHO/CDS/CPC/WHOPES/99.2) Geneva: World Health Organization.

1999b *Inventory of Applied Health Research in Emergency Settings.* Department of Emergency and Humanitarian Action. Geneva: World Health Organization.

2000a Severe falciparum malaria. *Transactions of the Royal Society of Tropical Medicine and Hygiene* 94(Suppl. 1):1-90.

2000b *Management of Severe Malaria: A Practical Handbook,* 2nd ed. Geneva: World Health Organization.

2001a New tools to roll back malaria. *Health in Emergencies* 9:4.

2001b *The Use of Antimalarial Drugs.: Report of an Informal Consultation.* (WHO/CDS/RBM/2001.33) Geneva: World Health Organization.

2002a International Travel and Health. Available: <*http://www.who.int/ith/index.html*> [September 25, 2002].

2002b *Monitoring Antimalarial Drug Resistance: Report of a WHO Consultation, March 5, 2001.* (WHO/CDS/RBM/2002.39) Geneva: World Health Organization.

Xiao, L., S.M. Owen, D.L. Rudolph, R.B. Lal, and A.A. Lal
1998 *Plasmodium falciparum* antigen-induced human immunodeficiency virus type 1 replication is mediated through induction of tumor necrosis factor-alpha. *Journal of Infectious Diseases* 177:437-445.

Young, H.
1999 Public nutrition in emergencies: An overview of debates, dilemmas and decision-making. *Disasters* 23:277-291.

Zetter, R.
1999 International perspectives on refugee assistance. Pp. 46-82 in *Refugees: Perspectives on the Experience of Forced Migration,* A. Ager, ed. London: Pinter.

Zucker, J.R.
1996 Changing patterns of autochthonous malaria transmission in the United States: A review of recent outbreaks. *Emerging Infectious Diseases* 2:37-43.

Appendix A

Description of Antimalarial Drugs

QUININE

Quinine was first isolated from Chinchona bark in 1820 and has since been the fundamental chemotherapeutic tool for the treatment of malaria, especially severe disease. Quinine and its dextroisomer, quinidine, are rapidly acting schizontocides that target the erythrocytic asexual stages of all malaria parasites. It is available in both oral and parenteral preparations and can be used in infants and pregnant women. Side effects include nausea, dysphoria, blurred vision, and tinnitus and typically resolve after treatment has ended. *P. falciparum* from most areas of the world responds well to quinine; thus, shortened courses of quinine can be used in conjunction with a second drug to reduce the likelihood of quinine-associated side effects. *P. falciparum* from many areas of Southeast Asia requires full-course quinine treatment in conjunction with a second drug (see Table 3-3), such as tetracycline.

CHLOROQUINE

Chloroquine is a 4-aminoquinoline derivative of quinine first synthesized in 1934. Historically, it has been the drug of choice for the treatment of nonsevere or uncomplicated malaria and for chemoprophylaxis. Chloroquine acts primarily against erythrocytic asexual stages, although it has gametocidal properties. Because of widespread resistance to this drug, its usefulness is increasingly limited. Where chloroquine retains efficacy it can be safely used for treatment or prophylaxis of infants and pregnant women. Side effects are uncommon and not generally serious. These include nausea, headache, gastrointestinal disturbance, and blurred vision. Some patients, especially if dark skinned, experience pruritus.

AMODIAQUINE

Amodiaquine is a drug closely related to chloroquine that fell out of favor because of a high incidence of adverse reactions (including agranulocytosis and hepatitis), primarily when used for prophylaxis, and drug resistance patterns similar to chloroquine. This drug is currently being reevaluated, especially as a possible component in artesunate-containing combination-therapy regimens. Concern over toxicity remains, however.

ANTIFOL COMBINATION DRUGS

These drugs are various combinations of dihydrofolate reductase inhibitors (proguanil, chlorproguanil, pyrimethamine, and trimethoprim) and sulfa drugs (dapsone, sulfalene, sulfamethoxazole, sulfadoxine, and others). Although these drugs have antimalarial activity when used alone, parasitological resistance can develop rapidly. When used in combination, they produce a synergistic effect on the parasite and can be effective even in the presence of resistance to the individual components. Typical combinations include sulfadoxine/pyrimethamine (Fansidar), sulfalene/pyrimethamine (Metakelfin), and sulfamethoxazole/trimethoprim (cotrimoxazole). Proguanil is often used in combination with chloroquine for prophylaxis in areas of moderate chloroquine resistance, although studies suggest that minimal additional benefit is derived, especially with prolonged exposure (Lobel et al., 1993; Steffen et al., 1993). Side effects are uncommon; however, severe allergic reactions can occur. When used prophylactically among American travelers, sulfadoxine/pyrimethamine has been associated with a high incidence of severe cutaneous reactions (1 per 5,000 to 8,000 users) and mortality (1 per 11,000 to 25,000 users; Miller et al., 1986). These side effects do not appear to occur as frequently when the drug is used for treatment. Concerns about sulfa drug use during pregnancy are outweighed by the known risks to mother and fetus of untreated malaria. Finally, use of folate supplementation concurrently with antifol antimalarials may increase the frequency of treatment failure (van Hensbroek et al., 1995).

Another promising antifol combination, chlorproguanil and dapsone, is currently being tested in Africa and elsewhere. Also known as "LapDap," this particular combination is innately more effective than sulfadoxine/pyrimethamine (even in areas where resistance is present) and also has a much shorter elimination half-life, which may decrease the chances for development of resistance (Watkins et al., 1997; Mutabingwa et al., 2001). Conversely, the shorter half-life requires that it be given over 3 days rather than in a single dose.

TETRACYCLINES

Tetracycline and derivatives such as doxycycline are very potent antimalarials and are used for either treatment or prophylaxis. In areas where response to quinine has deteriorated, tetracyclines are often used in combination with quinine to improve cure rates. Tetracyclines are also used in conjunction with shortened courses of quinine to decrease the likelihood of quinine-associated side effects (provided parasites are susceptible to quinine). Tetracyclines should not be used during pregnancy, breast-feeding, or in children under age 8. Common side effects include nausea, vomiting, diarrhea, *Candida* superinfections, and photosensitivity.

PRIMAQUINE

Primaquine, an 8-aminoquinoline, is primarily used as a tissue schizonticide for the purpose of reducing the likelihood of relapse due to hypnozoites of *P. vivax* and *P. ovale*. Studies have shown that primaquine has reasonably good efficacy (74 percent against *P. falciparum* and 90 percent against *P. vivax*) when used for prophylaxis (Baird et al., 1995). Although it has activity against blood-stage asexual parasites, the concentrations required to achieve blood schizonticidal action are toxic; primaquine is also a potent gametocidal drug. People with glucose-6-phosphate dehydrogenase (G6PD) deficiencies can experience severe and potentially fatal hemolytic anemia if treated with primaquine. The most severe Mediterranean B variant and related Asian variants of G6PD deficiency can occur at high rates among some groups and in some regions; Kurdish Jews (62 percent), Saudi Arabia (13 percent), Myanmar (20 percent), and southern China (6 percent). Migration, mutation, and intermarriage have spread these variants throughout the world. Primaquine should not be used in pregnancy.

Tafenoquine, a synthetic primaquine analog, is currently being tested. It is highly effective against both liver and blood stages of malaria. Because of its long half-life (14 days versus 6 hours for primaquine), tafenoquine may prove to be a valuable chemoprophylactic drug (Lell et al., 2000). As for primaquine, tafenoquine can result in hemolysis among patients with G6PD deficiency.

MEFLOQUINE

Mefloquine is a quinoline-methanol derivative of quinine. Mefloquine can be used either therapeutically or prophylactically in most areas with multidrug-resistant malaria. Resistance to mefloquine, however, occurs frequently in parts of Southeast Asia; sporadic resistance has been reported in areas of Africa and South America. Mefloquine has been associated with a relatively high incidence of neuropsychiatric side effects when used at treatment doses but is otherwise well tolerated. Although not licensed for use during pregnancy and in very young infants, mefloquine appears to be safe and effective in both groups.

HALOFANTRINE

Halofantrine is a phenanthrene-methanol compound with activity against the erythrocytic stages of the malaria parasite. Its use has been especially recommended in areas with multidrug-resistant falciparum. Studies have indicated, however, that the drug can produce cardiac conduction abnormalities (specifically, prolongation of the PR and QT interval[1]), limiting its usefulness (Nosten et al., 1993). A subsequent study suggests that cardiac abnormalities are dose dependent and can be severe in patients with preexisting cardiopathy; the authors suggest that electrocardiography be conducted on all patients prior to treatment with halofantrine (Monlun et al., 1995). A micronized formulation has improved halofantrine's poor oral bioavailability; however, it should be given on an empty stomach. Fatty foods dramatically increase absorption, increasing the risk of cardiac complications. Recrudescences can occur with one round of treatment, and, especially when treating nonimmune individuals, a second course should

---

[1]PR and QT intervals are specific points on an electrocardiogram. They are the intervals between the P and R wave forms and between the Q and T wave forms, respectively.

be given 7 days later. Retreatment of patients who had failed mefloquine therapy with halofantrine was less successful than primary treatment with halofantrine, suggesting the possibility of clinical cross-resistance between the two drugs (Wongsrichanalai et al., 1992; ter Kuile et al., 1993). Halofantrine therapy after mefloquine or quinine therapy also increases the risk of cardiac problems.

CLINDAMYCIN

Clindamycin has some antimalarial activity but is a poor choice compared to the other available antimalarial drugs. It is a slow-acting schizonticide and should only be used in combination with a fast-acting schizonticide, such as quinine, especially when treating patients with little or no immunity to malaria (Pukrittayakamee et al., 2000b; Parola et al., 2001). Although clindamycin may be useful for treatment of pregnant women and very young children (Pukrittayakamee et al., 2000a) more effective drugs are available that can be used in these groups (such as mefloquine or even, perhaps, mefloquine + artesunate).

ARTEMISININ COMPOUNDS

A number of sesquiterpine lactone compounds have been synthesized from the plant *Artemisia annua* (artesunate, artemether, artether). Benefits of use for severe malaria include rapid parasite clearance times and faster fever resolution than occurs with quinine. Preliminary results of studies to determine if this faster action produces improved survival suggest that there is quicker improvement of coma following treatment with artemisinins (Taylor et al., 1993; Salako et al., 1994). When used alone, especially for durations of less than 5 to 7 days, recrudescence rates are high. For nonsevere malaria, artemisinins are most successfully used in combination with a second drug (Nosten et al., 1994a). The best-documented combination therapy is that using mefloquine and 3 days of artesunate.

A fixed-dose preparation of lumefantrine and artemether is commercially available (Co-artem or Riamet). Lumefantrine (previously known as benflumetol) is an aryl-amino alcohol antimalarial compound. Although related chemically, in practice, lumefantrine does not appear to have cardiac effects similar to halofantrine (van Vugt et al., 1999). This combination is marketed in two packaging schemes: a six-dose (24-tablet) package for use by nonimmune patients, and a four-dose (16-tablet) package for use by semiimmune patients. Until studies have conclusively shown adequate efficacy of the four-dose regimen among semiimmune populations, all patients should probably be treated with a full six-dose regimen (van Vugt et al., 2000). No data exist to prove the safety of lumefantrine use during pregnancy; thus, lumefantrine should not be used to treat pregnant women.

ATOVAQUONE PLUS PROGUANIL (MALARONE)

This drug is a fixed-dose antimalarial combination of 250 mg of atovaquone and 100 mg of proguanil. Atovaquone is a hydroxynaptho-quinone that is currently being used mostly to treat opportunistic infections in immunosuppressed patients. Because of a high incidence of recrudescence when used alone, atovaquone is given in combination with proguanil (Looareesuwan et al., 1996a; Radloff et al., 1996). Treatment is with 1,000 mg of atovaquone and 400 mg of proguanil daily for 3 days. Malarone is reportedly effective against erythrocytic forms of *P. vivax* (Looareesuwan et al., 1996a). Although there is some concern about resistance developing rapidly to this combination, Malarone currently appears to be highly effective against most drug-resistant malaria parasites.

PYRONARIDINE

Pyronaridine is a drug synthesized and used in China for over 20 years. While it was reportedly 100 percent effective in one trial in Cameroon, the drug was only 63 to 88 percent effective in Thailand (Ringwald et al., 1996; Looareesuwan et al., 1996b). Further testing is required before pyronaridine can be recommended for use.

APPENDIX B

Methodology for Efficacy Assessment of In Vivo Malaria Therapy

INTRODUCTION

A standardized protocol for assessing antimalarial drug efficacy in vivo is available from the World Health Organization (1996c, 2002b) and should be used wherever possible. The following is a brief description of the protocol.

METHODS

Patients presenting to a health clinic with fever or history of fever suggestive of malaria are evaluated with thick blood smears for inclusion. In areas where malaria is highly endemic and acquired immunity is likely to be high, patients should be limited to those in the highest-risk groups (i.e., children less than 5 years of age). In areas where malaria is less intensely transmitted and acquired immunity is likely to be low, all age groups are at risk of clinical illness and are appropriate participants. Those who have a parasite density above a defined level are treated with a standard dose of antimalarial drug under supervision to ensure compliance. Follow-up thick blood smears are typically obtained on days 2 and 3, 7 days after initiation of treatment, and then once every 7 days for the duration of follow-up. The duration of posttreatment follow-up depends on the malaria transmission level (and therefore the probability that reappearance of malaria parasites could be due to reinfection instead of drug failure), the drug being used, and the likelihood of good follow-up success. In sub-Saharan Africa, 14 days of follow-up is recommended in most situations. In areas with low transmission, a follow-up period of 28 days or longer might be more appropriate. In some cases a 7-day follow-up period has been used, although this would likely underestimate failure rates, perhaps substantially. Patients are always encouraged to return to the clinic should symptoms recur between regularly scheduled visits. Every effort should be made to find patients not returning for scheduled visits. Failure to do this may seriously bias the results.

INTERPRETATION

Drug efficacy is best measured using both parasitological failure and clinical failure as outcomes. The World Health Organization has defined standard definitions for both parasitological failure and clinical failure. The definitions differ somewhat for areas with high transmission, with differences in the protocol highlighted for areas of low/moderate transmission. The definitions below are the ones applied to areas of high malaria transmission.

Classification of Response to Treatment

These are outcome measures based on changes in the patient's clinical condition in response to a standard dose of an antimalarial drug:

a. *Early treatment failure (ETF)*
   - Development of danger signs or severe malaria on Day 1, Day 2, or Day 3, in the presence of parasitemia **OR**
   - Parasitemia on Day 3 with axillary temperature greater than or equal to ($\geq$) 37.5°C **OR**
   - Parasitemia on Day 2 higher than Day 0 count
   - Parasitemia on Day 3 greater than or equal to ($\geq$) 25% of count on Day 0.

   NOTE: No differences for areas of low/moderate transmission.

b. *Late treatment failure (LTF)*
   b1. *Late clinical failure:*
   - Development of danger signs or severe malaria after Day 3 in the presence of parasitemia, without previously meeting any of the criteria of ETF **OR**

- Presence of parasitemia and axillary temperature greater than or equal to (≥) 37.5° on any day from Day 4 to Day 14,[1] without previously meeting any of the criteria for ETF.

  b2. *Late parasitologic failure:*

- Presence of parasitemia on Day 14[2] **AND** axillary temperature less than (<) 37.5°C, without previously meeting any of the criteria of ETF or late clinical failure.

c. *Adequate clinical and parasitological response (ACPR):*

- An absence of parasitemia on Day 14,[3] irrespective of axillary temperature, without previously meeting any of the criteria of early treatment failure or late clinical or parasitological failure.

NOTE
Parasitological Response

Parasitological response refers to the change in parasite density in response to a standard dose of an antimalarial drug. The parasitological response is categorized below.

There have been previous versions of the current recommended *in vivo* protocol and some readers may be more familiar with the definitions formally used to describe parasitological response. The terms RIII, RII, Early RI and Sensitive/Late RI are described below.[4]

---

[1]Day 4 to Day 28 in areas of low/moderate transmission.

[2]On any day from Day 7 to Day 28 in areas of low/moderate transmission.

[3]Absence of parasitemia on Day 28 in areas of low/moderate transmission.

[4]Previous versions of WHO (World Health Organization, 1996c) recommended *in vivo* methods used the "R system" to classify parasitological response. RIII denotes a severely resistant response in which little or no decline in parasite densities is observed within the first 48 to 72 hours posttreatment. RII denotes a moderately resistant response in which substantial declines in parasite density are observed within the first 48 to 72 hours posttreatment, but actual clearance does not occur and the patient continues to remain parasitemic through day 7 posttreatment. RI denotes a mildly resistant response in which parasitemia declines substantially within the first 48 to 72 hours posttreatment, is apparently cleared on subsequent examinations, but recrudesces sometime during follow-up. S denotes a fully sensitive response in which parasites are cleared and patients remain parasite free for the duration of follow-up. These tests and classification schemes were originally designed for follow-ups of at least 28 days. Studies using shorter follow-up periods (such as 14 days) are incapable of distinguishing an S response from a late RI response (i.e., parasites recrudesce between Day 14 and Day 28), so patients who remain parasite free for the 14-day follow-up period are often classified as S/RI. Actual definitions can be found in Bloland et al. (1993) as well as many other references.

a. RIII: a Day 2 parasite density that is greater than (>25) percent of the day 0 parasite density.

b. RII: a positive Day 2 blood smear with a parasite density that is less than or equal to (≤) 25 percent of the Day 0 density and a positive Day 7 blood smear.

c. Early RI: **EITHER**

- Negative Day 2 blood smear with a positive blood smear on any day between Day 3 and Day 14, **OR**
- Positive Day 2 blood smear with a parasite density that is less than (<) 25 percent of Day 0,
- Negative Day 7 blood smear,
- Positive blood smear on any day between Day 8 and Day 14.

d. Sensitive/Late RI

- A Day 2 parasite density that is less than (<) 25 percent of the Day 0 density **AND** negative blood smears on every follow-up examination between Day 7 and Day 14.

With follow-up periods of 14 days, it is not possible to distinguish sensitive responses from late recrudescences, and these responses are combined in the RI/S category. For follow-up periods longer than 14 days, the "late RI" definition is applied to any reappearance of parasites between Day 14 and the end of follow-up. "Sensitive" responses are reserved for those patients not experiencing reappearance of parasites for the duration of follow-up.

APPENDIX C

Alternative Treatment Regimens for Severe Malaria

The recommended treatment regimen for management of severe malaria given in Chapter 6 assumes that a fairly high level of patient care is possible (i.e., availability of intravenous therapy). There are clearly situations where this would not be the case. The following regimens allow for treatment of severe malaria in settings where such capacity is not available (World Health Organization, 2000a, 2000b).

Note: The use of suppositories containing an artemisinin drug is based on limited clinical experience but is the subject of ongoing clinical trials.

INTRAMUSCULAR QUININE

Loading Dose

Quinine dihydrochloride is given intramuscularly at 20 mg salt/kg diluted to 60 mg/ml in normal saline. The dose should be split between two injection sites in the anterior thigh (not the buttocks).

Maintenance Dose

Eight hours after the loading dose, quinine dihydrochloride is given intramuscularly at 10 mg salt/kg and repeated every 8 hours until the patient can take oral medication. Oral medication should follow the regimen described in Chapter 6.

INTRAMUSCULAR ARTEMISININ DRUGS

Artesunate can be given intramuscularly at 2.4 mg/kg initially, followed by 1.2 mg/kg 12 hours and 24 hours later, then 1.2 mg/kg daily for 6 days. An oral artemisinin compound can be used once the patient can take oral medication. Alternatively, after a minimum of 3 days of artesunate, patients able to take oral medications can be switched to another antimalarial drug appropriate to the area (e.g., either sulfadoxine/pyrimethamine or mefloquine in areas where those drugs remain effective).

Artemether can be given intramuscularly at 3.2 mg/kg on the first day, followed by 1.6 mg/kg daily for 6 days. An oral artemisinin compound can be used once the patient can take oral medication. Alternatively, after a minimum of 3 days of artesunate, patients able to take oral medications can be switched to another antimalarial drug appropriate to the area (e.g., either sulfadoxine/pyrimethamine or mefloquine in areas where those drugs remain effective).

INTRARECTAL ARTEMISININ DRUGS

Artemisinin suppositories can be given using a 40 mg/kg loading dose, followed by 20 mg/kg at 4, 24, 48, and 72 hours. Patients able to take oral medications can then be switched to an oral artemisinin drug at an appropriate dose or another antimalarial drug appropriate to the area (e.g., either sulfadoxine/pyrimethamine or mefloquine in areas where those drugs remain effective).

Artesunate suppositories can be given using one 200-mg suppository initially, followed by one 200-mg suppository at 12, 24, 36, 48, and 60 hours. Patients able to take oral medications can then be switched to an oral artemisinin drug at an appropriate dose or another antimalarial drug appropriate to the area (e.g., either sulfadoxine/pyrimethamine or mefloquine in areas where those drugs remain effective).

For additional details and recommendations, refer to World Health Organization (2000a, 2000b).

Appendix D

Malaria Research and Technical Resources

GENERAL INFORMATION

- World Health Organization/Roll Back Malaria (RBM) (*<http://www.rbm.who.int>*): RBM offers information and technical assistance for malaria control in complex emergencies. Listed below are examples of the types of resources available from the RBM website:

1. "Outline Strategy for Malaria Control in Complex Emergencies" (*<http://www.who.int/eha/resource/manuals/guidelines/malaria/rationale>*)
2. Malaria profiles of 20 affected countries.
3. Technical Resource Network (TRN): The TRN offers technical field support to affected countries, NGOs, and others requesting assistance. The coordinated field support generally lasts 2 weeks to 2 months. This partnership of experts includes representatives from the World Health Organization (WHO), the United Nations High Commissioner for Refugees (UNHCR), the United Nations Children's Fund (UNICEF), the Centers for Disease Control and Prevention (CDC), the International Federation of the Red Cross (IFRC), the Shoklo Malaria Research Unit (SMRU), the International Committee of the Red Cross (ICRC), Médecins Sans Frontières (MSF), MERLIN, HealthNet, and the Malaria Consortium. TRN contacts are given below:

1. Roll Back Malaria Tech Resource Network for Malaria Control in
   Complex Emergencies
   ATTN: Secretariat
   World Health Organization
   20, Avenue Appia
   CH 1211
   Geneva, Switzerland
   <http://mosquito.WHO.int>
   RBM Technical Strategies Malaria in Emergencies
2. Dr. Holly Ann Williams (point of contact for U.S.-based non-
   governmental organizations)
   Malaria Epidemiology Branch
   Centers for Disease Control and Prevention
   MS F-22
   4770 Buford Hwy NE
   Atlanta, GA 30341
   USA
   hbw2@cdc.gov
   (770) 488-7764

- *An Interagency Handbook on Malaria Control in Complex Emergencies*
(in press).
- World Health Organization

1. J.A. Nájera, R.L. Kouznetzsov, and C. Delacollette, *Malaria Epidemics: Detection and Control, Forecasting and Prevention,* WHO/
   MAL/98.1084, 1998.
2. J.A. Nájera, *Malaria Control Among Refugees and Displaced Populations,* CTD/MAL/96.6, WHO Division of Control of Tropical
   Diseases, Malaria Unit, 1996.
3. WHO, *WHO Expert Committee on Malaria (20th Report),* WHO
   Technical Report Series No. 892, 2000.
4. *Manual for Indoor Residual Spraying, Application of Residual Sprays
   for Vector Control,* WHO/CDS/WHOPES/GCDPP/2000.3, WHO
   Communicable Disease Control, Prevention and Eradication,
   WHO Pesticide Evaluation Scheme, 2000.

- Malaria Foundation International (*<http://www.malaria.org>*): The
foundation's mission is to facilitate the development and implementation
of solutions to the health, economic, and social problems caused by malaria.

- Multilateral Initiative on Malaria (MIM) (<*http://mim.nih.gov*>).
- NetMark (<*http://www.netmarkafrica.org*>): NetMark seeks an innovative approach to preventing malaria in Africa by promoting insecticide-treated materials (ITMs) through the formation of public-private partnerships.
- The Sphere Project (<*http://www.sphereproject.org*>): This project has developed a humanitarian charter and a set of universal minimum standards in core areas of humanitarian assistance: water supply and sanitation, nutrition, food aid, shelter and site planning, and health care services. The aim of the project is to improve the quality of assistance provided to people affected by disasters and to enhance the accountability of the humanitarian system in disaster response.

DIAGNOSTIC AIDS

- Centers for Disease Control and Prevention

1. DPDx: (<*http://www.dpd.cdc.gov/dpdx*>): A web-based program to assist in the identification of parasites of public health concern. DPDx (Division of Parasitic Diseases Diagnosis) offers two complimentary functions: a reference and training function and a diagnostic assistance function. For laboratories with such a capacity, digital images can be submitted via the Internet.

- World Health Organization:

1. *Bench Aids for the Diagnosis of Malaria (Plates No. 1-8)*, WHO, Geneva, 1999.
2. *Basic Malaria Microscopy (Part I: Learner's Guide, Part II: Tutor's Guide)*, WHO, Geneva, 1991.

CASE MANAGEMENT

- Severe malaria

1. World Health Organization, Severe falciparum malaria, *Transactions of the Royal Society of Tropical Medicine and Hygiene*, 94 (Suppl. 1), 2000.

2. World Health Organization, *Management of Severe Malaria: A Practical Handbook,* 2nd ed., WHO, Geneva, 2000. Also available at *<http://www.rbm.who.int.>*

3. J. Crawley. Reducing deaths from malaria among children: The pivotal role of prompt, effective treatment, *Africa Health* (Suppl., Sept. 25). Available via RBM website.

* Pregnancy

1. *Malaria in Pregnancy,* proceedings of a workshop held in Liverpool in September 1998 at the Second European Congress on Tropical Medicine, *Annals of Tropical Medicine and Parasitology,* 93 (Suppl. 1), Dec. 1999.

MISCELLANEOUS COMPLEX EMERGENCY AGENCIES AND PROGRAMS

* Johns Hopkins University, Refugee and Disaster Studies: *<http://jhspu.edu/Refugee/links.html>*
* Center of Excellence in Disaster Management and Humanitarian Assistance: *<http://website.tamc.amedd.army.mil>*
* University of Wisconsin-Disaster Management Center: *<http://epdwww.engr.wisc.edu/dmc>*
* UCLA Center for Public Health and Disaster Relief: *<http://www.ph.ucla/cphdr>*
* Refugee Studies Centre, Queen Elizabeth House, University of Oxford: *<http://www.qeh.ox.ac.uk/rsc>*. Offers an excellent documentation center and training programs.
* Columbia University Program on Forced Migration and Health: *<http://cpmcnet.columbia.edu/dept/sph/popfam/rp/forced_health>*
* Relief Web: *<http://www.reliefweb.int/w/rwb.nsf>*

RESEARCH TOOLS

* Catholic Relief Services (*<http://www.catholicrelief.org>*). Offers a resource manual on rapid and participatory research that can be used to conduct behavioral research in a complex emergency (*Rapid Rural Appraisal and Participatory Rural Appraisal Manual): <http://www.catholicrelief.org/what/overseas/rra_manual.cfm>*.

• Center for International Emergency, Disaster and Refugee Studies, Johns Hopkins Bloomberg School of Public Health: <*http://www.jhsph.edu/ refugee/resources.html*>. Offers resources for qualitative research methods.

TEXTS OF INTEREST

• Médecins Sans Frontières, *Refugee Health: An Approach to Emergency Situations,* Macmillan, London, 1997.
• H.M. Gilles and D.A. Warrell, *Bruce-Chwatt's Essential Malariology,* 3rd ed., Arnold, London, 1993.
• National Association of Practicing Anthropologists, *Caring for Those in Crisis: Integrating Anthropology and Public Health in Complex Humanitarian Emergencies,* NAPA Bulletin 21, American Anthropological Association, Washington, D.C., 2001. The issue is devoted to strengthening the ties between anthropology and public health practitioners, and malaria is used as an example in several chapters. For information on obtaining the bulletin: <*http://www.napabulletin.org/bulletin21.htm*>

APPENDIX E

About the Authors

Peter B. Bloland, an epidemiologist, is chief of the Case Management Activity in the Malaria Epidemiology Branch, Division of Parasitic Diseases, Centers for Disease Control and Prevention, Atlanta, Georgia. He received his Doctor of Veterinary Medicine and Masters in Preventive Veterinary Medicine degrees from the University of California at Davis. He is a member of the Roll Back Malaria Technical Resource Network on Malaria Control in Complex Emergencies. His refugee field experience includes Zaire, Eritrea, and Tanzania. He has published papers in *Lancet* and *Refuge* regarding complex emergencies, in *Caring for Those in Crisis: Integrating Anthropology and Public Health in Complex Humanitarian Emergencies* (2001, the National Association for Practicing Anthropologists [NAPA] Bulletin 21), and is a contributing author to an interagency handbook on malaria control in the context of complex emergencies, being published by UNCHR and WHO. His current research interests in regard to complex emergencies include general malaria control and prevention and antimalarial drug resistance.

Holly Ann Williams is an anthropologist assigned to the Case Management Activity within the Malaria Epidemiology Branch, Division of Parasitic Diseases, Centers for Disease Control and Prevention, Atlanta, Georgia. She received her Ph.D. in medical and cultural anthropology from the University of Florida and has a clinical specialty in pediatric nursing, with a Masters in Nursing degree from the University of Washington.

The **Committee on Population** was established by the National Academy of Sciences (NAS) in 1983 to bring the knowledge and methods of the population sciences to bear on major issues of science and public policy. The committee's work includes both basic studies of fertility, health and mortality, and migration; and applied studies aimed at improving programs for the public health and welfare in the United States and in developing countries. The committee also fosters communication among researchers in different disciplines and countries and policy makers in government and international agencies.

The **Roundtable on the Demography of Forced Migration** was established by the Committee on Population of the National Academy of Sciences in 1999. The Roundtable's purpose is to serve as an interdisciplinary, nonpartisan focal point for taking stock of what is known about demographic patterns in refugee situations, applying this knowledge base to assist both policy makers and relief workers, and stimulating new directions for innovation and scientific inquiry in this growing field of study. The Roundtable meets yearly and has also organized a series of workshops (held concurrently with Roundtable meetings) on some of the specific aspects of the demography of refugee and refugee-like situations, including mortality patterns, demographic assessment techniques, and research ethics in complex humanitarian emergencies. The Roundtable is composed of experts from academia, government, philanthrophy, and international organizations.

Other Publications of the Roundtable on the Demography of Forced Migration

Research Ethics in Complex Humanitarian Emergencies: Summary of a Workshop (2002)
Demographic Assessment Techniques in Complex Humanitarian Emergencies: Summary of a Workshop (2002)
Forced Migration and Mortality (2001)

During 1988, she was a study fellow in the Refugee Studies Programme at Oxford University, England. She is a member of the American Anthropological Association's Committee on Refugee and Immigrants (CORI). She has public health, clinical, and research experience in Thailand, Sudan, Tanzania, and Zambia, working with refugees in camps, self-settled refugees and internally displaced persons. She is also a member of the Roll Back Malaria Technical Resource Network on Malaria Control in Complex Emergencies and is a contributing author to an interagency handbook on malaria control in the context of complex emergencies, being published by UNCHR and WHO. She has authored or coauthored papers relating to refugee studies in the journals *Human Organization*, and *Refuge,* as well as the edited volume *Selected Papers on Refugee Issues: Volume II* (American Anthropology Association). In addition, she served as editor for *Caring for Those in Crisis: Integrating Anthropology and Public Health in Complex Humanitarian Emergencies* (2001, the National Association for Practicing Anthropologists [NAPA] Bulletin 21). Currently, her research interests include malaria control in complex emergencies, the formulation and implementation of national antimalarial drug treatment policies, and sociobehavioral issues related to malaria control.